Learning Curves

Learning Curves

Helen Gaize

Matador
9 Priory Business Park,
Wistow Road, Kibworth Beauchamp,
Leicestershire. LE8 0RX
Tel: 0116 279 2299
Email: books@troubador.co.uk
Web: www.troubador.co.uk/matador
Twitter: @matadorbooks

ISBN 978 1784625 504

British Library Cataloguing in Publication Data.
A catalogue record for this book is available from the British Library.

Printed and bound in the UK by TJ International, Padstow, Cornwall
Typeset in 11pt Aldine401 BT by Troubador Publishing Ltd, Leicester, UK

Matador is an imprint of Troubador Publishing Ltd

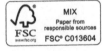

CONTENTS

FOREWORD

The events described in this book began fifteen years ago. During the ensuing years, I know that many aspects of treatment and practice will have changed or improved. Fifteen years is a very long learning time in terms of the treatment of cancer and in the world of plastic surgery. However, I can only tell my own story, and that is what I have set down here for you. It is important to state that, for most people, the journey from diagnosis to discharge, even then, was very much less complicated, and very much swifter, than mine – but I can only write from my own experience. I am, in any case, delighted with my positive outcome!

As is often the case in this genre of writing, some names of persons and locations in my account have been changed in order to protect the privacy and rights of others.

I owe huge thanks to all of the surgical, medical and hospital personnel, without exception, who were so patient with me and my trials and demands. They not only saved my life but quite literally made me the person I physically am today, and that was some task!

Huge thanks are due also to Professor Jane Plant for her wonderful book, 'Your Life in Your Hands', indispensable, in my view, as it is so very helpful to those suffering from breast cancer. She has books to help those diagnosed with other cancers also.

Those who are affected by Life and fertility issues similar to the ones described in these pages can now find a rich source of information and help from the website of NaPro TECHNOLOGY and the work of Thomas W Hilgers, MD, whose definitive textbook was published in 2004.

The many people who accompanied me on my journey and as I wrote know who they are: they are too numerous to name. They also know that I will never be able to thank them enough for all that they have done for me. Without their support I would have been lost. I am particularly blessed in my family; thank-you all.

Most importantly, and always... Glory be to the Father, and to the Son, and to the Holy Spirit, as it was in the beginning, is now, and ever shall be! Thank-you, God! Amen.

Part One

Learning Curves

and

Pearls

I had done everything right. That was what made the whole situation somehow harder to grasp. Mum had died of breast cancer when I was thirty. I had attended for regular mammograms since. I had been 'breast aware'. A couple of lumps had been removed and investigated as a precaution; they were benign.

Self-examination of my breasts had always been difficult. Due to that surgery, and also to fertility treatment I had received in my twenties, they were always 'lumpy'. They were also large – a size 34 G or H cup – which no one outside an unhealthy media spotlight could possibly desire! Indeed, I would have qualified for breast reduction surgery on the NHS, had I sought it, due to the damage caused by the weight of the bra straps on my shoulders. However, I had done my best. Throughout the period of my cancer treatment, I found this rankled with me more and more: I had a powerful feeling that, despite everybody's best efforts, the system had somehow let me down. After all, we are continually told of the importance of early detection, yet, despite everything, my tumour had obviously had plenty of time to become established…

As I undressed one warm evening in late April I noticed that there was a really appreciable impression of the seaming of my bra on an area of my lower left breast. The area seemed swollen, as if lymphatic flow had been impeded: as if that clear fluid that travels round our bodies and is part of our means of fighting infection had somehow got dammed up in my breast. I told myself that the day had been hot and everything would look better in the morning. It did. Better, but not right. The skin appeared thicker there when pinched too, and try as I might, I could not make the skin of the right breast appear the same. I waited about a week. This was not going to resolve. I made an appointment to see the doctor.

In common with most General Practice clinics these days, at mine there was usually a long waiting list to see the doctor on whose list you were registered, but it was possible to be seen by the duty doctor in the practice as an 'emergency' within a day or two. That was the option I selected and I saw, late and tired one evening, a very experienced male doctor who had been with the practice for years. It had obviously been a very long day for him. I could see the weariness in his face as I launched into my 'I'm sorry if I'm bothering you for nothing, but...' routine. I think he truly thought I was. He was very kind, examined my breasts, pronounced that the states of right and left were pretty similar as far as he could see, agreed that they were large and difficult to examine and told me, to my immense relief, that he thought I had nothing to worry about. I went home so happy!

The euphoria was short-lived. Soon I was showing the area of concern to one of my closest female friends, who happens to be a nurse and midwife and has seen a lot of breasts in her time. She pronounced the breast definitely oedematous, swollen with fluid. I knew she would. I knew it was. This was just not right and it wasn't going away. I had to do something.

About three weeks after the doctor had given me the all clear I contacted the Breast Care Clinic. I made an appointment for a consultation myself, and this was only possible because I was already registered as a patient there due to my regular mammograms. I was not due to be seen by them until the following November, but the appointment was brought forward at my request because I felt I had noted significant changes. I had last been examined the previous November, and this is interesting because, as I understand it, the cancer must have been present at that time, yet it had not shown on the mammogram and I had been given an all clear for the next twelve months. Now, five months later, I was sure that I was detecting something alarming that the medics had so far missed.

It is important at this point to state that I was in a very fortunate position here. Most women would not have had access to the clinic as it is necessary to be referred there by a GP. Since I was already registered I did not need a re-referral, but remember that the GP I had seen had not thought it necessary to take the matter any further. I do not doubt his good faith or his healing intentions, but I am so glad that I was able to seek further help for myself and I did not have to wait until November.

I was seen at the end of the first week of June. On that very first visit a consultant with a heart of gold, who whirls around the hospital abrading the floors with his shoe leather, mobilised everyone in his power on my behalf and achieved a mammogram and an ultrasound scan for me, both without appointment, a normally impossible feat. Both were inconclusive, but he felt that there was a problem to be solved and made an appointment for me to see the head man in the team the following week. In fact, I owe an awful lot to the kind doctor who, I think, had given up part of his lunch hour to do my ultrasound scan. At some point during that week, as I understand it, he held a magnifying glass over the x-ray film from the mammogram and identified calcium deposits. The kind consultant, when informed of these findings, rang my husband and suggested that I should have a biopsy at my next appointment in order to look more closely at these, rather than seeing his chief.

So it was that one week after the first appointment I turned up for minor surgery. Right from the start, a phrase had to be used that I learned to hate, because I have heard it so often and in so many contexts since all this began. 'Normally we…but in your case…' The problem was always the size of my breasts. The quest for samples of the calcium deposits was described as searching for a needle in a haystack. I was really very fortunate, however, because our local breast unit is one of the best in the country, and the level of treatment offered to ladies in my position is often very much a lottery. I know that, since that first consultation, I have had the very best that those who worked on my case could offer and this is largely due to the dedication of the staff, though up-to-date equipment is a very positive bonus.

My left breast was clamped between plates as for a mammogram and I realised that, once again, I was to be exposed to x-rays in order for the treatment to take place. In these days when babes in the womb are so often considered disposable, this doesn't always seem to be a major issue to the medical establishment (though women who know they are pregnant are asked to inform radiographers, little attention seems to be paid to the possibility of an early unplanned, unknown pregnancy) but if there *was* a tiny life at stake, it was a very important issue to me – and according to my belief, to the God who put it there. This would be my second x-ray in eight days. Before the emergency mammogram the preceding week, I had to shoot into town and buy a pregnancy test. The hospital had been unable to supply one and unwilling to proceed with the examination without the result of one because I could not sign a declaration that I was not pregnant.

My husband and I did not use contraception – why would we, when we spent much of our early married life on fertility treatment? I have been pregnant three times and never carried to term. We have two wonderful adopted children, the children not of our bodies but of our hearts – but if God had chosen to send us another late in life, we would not have wanted to close doors! So now, once again, there was great debate. Finally, the good doctor said that had I been his mother or his sister, he would have urged me strongly to proceed with the examination, and on the strength of that, a lead apron was produced, wrapped around my abdomen, and we were away!

'Normally, we take five or so samples, but you have been very good because we have had to take fifteen to be sure that we have what we're looking for.' The doctor was kind, gentle and thorough, and the nurses generous afterwards with hot chocolate to drink and a large, fancy, chocolate sweet to eat. I had been 'clamped in' for about an hour and was trembling with shock when I came out. I needed blood sugar, and I was sore. I teach, and that evening was to be a particularly gruelling parents' evening. I went. Somehow, the routine has to go on. I just drank a lot of sweetened tea.

Looking back, I wonder if I would do such a thing again. The biopsy, almost always relatively quick and painless, had, because of the size of my breast, undoubtedly been very traumatic. After it, I really had been in a state of shock. Behaving as most conscientious workers would in the circumstances, it had not really occurred to me to just go home and rest; I felt my responsibilities to my job too keenly. Yet when I recall how I was feeling and how very sore I was, it seems to me now like some kind of madness. We in the West have grown too accustomed to the work ethic. Society seems to divide itself between those who feel at ease taking sick leave as a form of time out and those who find it very difficult indeed to draw a demarcation line between their duty of work and the rest of their lives, frequently to the detriment of themselves and maybe their loved ones. At the time, I fell into the latter camp, but I am beginning, rather late, to learn the meaning of, 'To everything there is a season and a time for every purpose under Heaven'.

In fact, the machine used for my biopsies had been a very clever one, capable of taking selected core samples from my breast, at various depths, through a rectangular hole in the top plate of the clamp. This was all achieved, without pain during the procedure, under local anaesthetic. Sitting clamped in this fashion for such a length of time had indeed been gruelling and far from comfortable, but every effort had been made at all times to put me as much at ease as possible. With all fifteen cores successfully extracted, the doctor had assured me with a grin that I would definitely have lost weight! The results of the biopsies would be known in a week.

Exactly one week later, I was in one of a row of examination rooms, once again naked from the waist up, and waiting to see the head man, the top consultant. He too is a man of dedication. He has a well-deserved reputation and really knows his stuff. He entered the room, stood reading my file at the window ledge, drumming his fingers the while: then he turned to me and said, 'You have a problem in your breast, my dear.' And that was it. I had cancer. When the good biopsy doctor had shown me, under the magnifying glass, the features he was going after the week before, I had said, 'It looks like the Milky Way.' It had been purely an observation based on the way the calcium dots appeared to me, like the constellation of that name. The doctor had shot me a strange look but said nothing. Now the big chief was explaining these deposits to me, and I once again used the term. He was taken aback and told me that that was the correct clinical term used to describe the feature. The deposits were laid down by the progressing cancer and provided the means to detect it.

My husband's face was stricken. I told him that there was no point at all in coming to a place like the clinic to be monitored for ominous changes if we were going to become distressed when they found some. Wasn't that what it was all about? The consultant was encouraging – a wide local excision to remove the primary and a goodly area of tissue around it; a lymphectomy (removal of some or all of my lymph nodes under my arm) to check that the disease had not invaded my lymph glands; some radiotherapy to put the brakes on any seed-bed area in the breast threatening future development... I asked him how I was going to tell my father.

Not only had my mother died of breast cancer, but when my father remarried, his second wife, my stepmother, had also suffered from the disease. True, she had recovered and had since died of entirely unrelated causes, but Dad was not going to find a third bite at this cherry easy! The consultant suggested there would be no need to tell him. It seemed likely that, if I came in the next week for surgery, the whole episode might well be closed, done and dusted in a matter of months. Although I knew I would have to be honest with Dad, I took this as a very encouraging scenario from the main man and was grateful.

At our centre, when a consultant is going to give you the kind of news I had just received, one of two breast care nurses is called in. These two ladies are particularly dedicated. They are there to hear what the specialist says and to make sure that the patient understands and does not miss important information due to shock. After the consultation, the nurse led me to another room. She went over the details of what I had been told very gently with me. We discussed what I should say to my children, in their late teens at this time; on the basis of the consultant's advice about my father, we decided that I would explain exactly what was to happen. Abnormal cells would be cut out of my breast, with a surrounding area of healthy tissue, and the breast would be treated to prevent a recurrence. I simply wouldn't use the word 'cancer' as this may be unduly alarming at this stage.

During this interview with the breast care nurse, patients are invariably given a very helpful Filofax, full of information on breast cancer and its treatment. It does seem a bit like, 'The bad news is you have breast cancer; the good news is you get the swanky Filofax,' but the intention and the information are both good. I clutched my copy, listened to the gentle advice about not reading bits yet that might never apply to me, such as the passages on chemotherapy, and tearfully asked questions.

I am a keen amateur guitarist. One of my chief pleasures is to play regularly, though not too professionally, in Christian music ministry. I knew from information that I had been given, that the removal of my lymph glands would put me at significant risk of lymph oedema, a swelling of the arm on the involved side due to the interruption of the lymph drainage, caused by surgery. One fifth of all women having such surgery experience this problem to a significant degree. Would I still be able to play? The answer was a resounding 'yes', but I was told that it might be necessary for me to wear an elastic sleeve to keep the swelling down.

Also, in common with all post-operative patients, I would be required to take Tamoxifen, a drug which lowers oestrogen levels. Breast tumours are often oestrogen or progestogen dependent, and our bodies make these hormones which feed our tumours. Tamoxifen helps to prevent that, but the thought of taking it frightened me because my mother had had to take it and she had attributed the loss of her singing voice to the action of this drug. I loved to sing. Would I be able to? Yes, but my range might change. Great!

I left the interview somewhat shell-shocked, but the nurse thoughtfully provided me with a telephone number so that, when I had had time to think, I could contact her at need with any questions. I have lost count of the number of times I dialled that number, yet I always found a helpful and sympathetic ear on the other end of the line.

For best part of a week, I worked as much as I felt able. The headmaster of the school where I teach was, throughout my sickness, exemplary in his support and the level of empathy he strove to achieve. I attended a pre-admission clinic on the Tuesday of the following week at the outpatients' department. On this day, I was counselled about what to expect from the surgery, what I would need in hospital, what the likely follow-up might be and so on. Blood tests were taken and I had yet another x-ray (yet another discussion, yet another lead apron), this time a general chest x-ray, in order to determine my fitness to undergo surgery. Once all the necessary information had been taken, the tests done and the counselling completed, we headed for home. It was about two in the afternoon. I would be admitted to hospital at about ten the next morning.

The hospital was genuinely welcoming. I was to have a bed in a four-bed side ward and I had no need to undress until the doctors needed to see me. My husband was encouraged to be with me as much as he could and was made very welcome in his own right. I was allowed visitors from two until eight, but I discovered that, if I needed company at other times, staff members were very flexible, understanding and accommodating. Obviously, it would not have been reasonable had my visitors disturbed other patients. Mutual consideration and respect are key issues.

Once I had been duly processed, I was marked up for the next morning's surgery with an indelible black marker pen; an asterisk on my left hand in order to ensure the correct side of me was being tackled, and a great arrow on my chest, pointing to the left breast. I had my hospital arm and leg bands for identification, and additional ones in red, giving information about my drug allergies. I met other, cheerful women whose stories were the same as, or similar to, my own. In a place such as this, the barriers come down. Lives outside are on hold and thrown here together, we forged a special bond. We ate together in a communal dining room, and retired early and chattily to bed. Most of us were, of course, breast patients as this was a specialist breast unit; however any bed space not required for breast patients held general surgical overspill. I slept well, and had opted to be woken in the night for an early breakfast of tea and toast. I felt it would help guard against sickness after the general anaesthetic.

I was taken to theatre in good spirits. I felt very confident in the abilities of my surgeon, and he was very much in evidence and very cheerful. The anaesthetist's assistant was a law student, working his holidays and hoping to specialise in medical litigation at the close of his studies. He was a striking young man with a cheeky and flirtatious manner. He even jocularly propositioned me! I had been accompanied to theatre by a student nurse who had asked permission to be present to witness my operation, and she was now wearing 'scrubs'. As they went gently about the process of anaesthetising me, I remember suggesting to her that she should remind her anaesthetist colleague to take care of his real self as well as the charming 'lady killing' persona that he, in his youth and confidence, was presenting to the world! I doubt if he took me seriously. At any rate I was grateful for his easy and relaxed manner, if a little concerned for his spiritual well-being!

Up to that point, preparation for theatre had been something of a stripping exercise. I was accustomed to wearing make-up, which of course is not allowed. I always wore certain jewellery, which was, in its way, my trade-mark. All of this had to go and it felt like losing my identity... I took off a treble clef on a chain, symbol of the Christian music ministry; a cross, the emblem of my faith; a garnet ring which was a gift from my husband; a wish-bone ring bought for me by my children; a Claddagh ring which was a gift from my closest friends; a 'mizpah' ring inherited from my father, and a signet ring handed on to me by my mother one birthday when I was still quite young. There was also my wedding ring, of course. This I was allowed to keep once it had been taped.

It felt as if these things helped to define me and with them about my person, I was somehow 'safe'. These things showed who I was, what I did, what I stood for...and only my wedding ring could go with me to theatre; my only physical treasure: 'Where your treasure is, there will your heart be also'. In addition, my daughter has always told me that, as far as she can see, the only redeeming factor in what she considers to be my appalling taste in summer sandals is the fact that I wear good polish on my fairly presentable toe-nails. Even that had to go. I was allowed to keep my briefs, but attired in a theatre gown and white socks to prevent thrombosis, I felt unattractive and vulnerable. Now I was stripped down to the 'me' which only I and God knew. It was definitely a 'Here we go, Lord,' moment... Him and me...

The surgery went very well and the surgeon was kind enough to come and see me afterwards to say so. He was confident that, having made an extra wide excision, the likelihood was that he had indeed 'got it all', though of course only the histology report, due in two weeks' time, could confirm that. I was returned to the ward. However, I had woken from the anaesthetic in tremendous pain. Normally this does not happen. It certainly did not happen in subsequent surgery I have experienced, and the fact that it happened to me should not alarm others, but I mention it because the team worked so very hard to relieve that pain. The most likely explanation is that one of the two drains in the wound was sited where it was drawing upon a nerve as it removed excess fluid from the surgery site. All I know is that the pain was so intense that I was reduced to tears, distressing my husband and alarming my son when they visited. The nurses were most concerned and contacted the consultant. He himself came to see me, suggested a new way of taping the drain in place and prescribed effective pain killing medication which was administered without delay. The relief was wonderful. I was able to relax and drowse and I began to luxuriate in the sensation of being sleepy and pain free, knowing the surgery was over.

It is a source of wonder to me that God can make good use of us even when we are at our weakest! That night, a lady was admitted to the opposite bed in acute pain caused by a chronic condition she suffered. She was put into our ward because this was where a bed was vacant and she frequently moaned or cried out in her discomfort. She had a paralysis of her lower body which deprived her of the use of her legs and made it very difficult for her to adjust her position in the bed and get comfortable. In particular, because of her acute pain and limited movement, though she often needed the help of a nurse, she could rarely reach the call button. Throughout that night, as I drifted in and out of sleep, I was aware of her distress and, at little cost to myself, able to be of service to her, calling the nurse when she could not, and talking to her to reassure her that someone else was awake and she was not alone. I slipped into sleep easily between times, thanks to the half-life of the anaesthetic and the pain-killing medication. Finally, her discomfort was eased and she was able to sleep. She was moved to another ward the next day.

There was also a young woman in the same side ward as me who, from the moment of my admission, proved to be a joy. I was so inspired by her courage. She had come to England from China, and her husband, also Chinese, worked locally and visited frequently with their gorgeous baby daughter, less than a year old. This young woman, Xiao Yan, had waited five years for her surgery, and had to have surgery to both underarm areas. Consequently she was in a lot of pain and had to cope with the drains that had been inserted into both sides of her body. She spoke almost no English, though she understood a little, so the whole experience of being in the hospital must have been very alarming indeed for her – everything from choosing food for the next day to receiving treatment without fully understanding it – yet she remained brave and cheerful and I was drawn to her. At first we communicated with the aid of hastily scribbled pictures, but we graduated to a stilted form of language with signs and gestures thrown in for good measure. Through visiting times we got to know each other's close family members and at mealtimes we kept each other company. I really valued her friendship and cheerful demeanour then and I still do now.

Given this situation, it was perhaps no accident that my Malaysian-Chinese friend, May, turned up to see me. She and Xiao Yan experienced an instant rapport. May was able to help Xiao Yan to understand better what was going on while she was in the hospital and the three of us have shared many good times since in Xiao Yan's home and mine. Had I not been in that ward at that time, May and Xiao Yan would not have met. God knows what He is about.

Recovering from my surgery took time. My intellect knew it would and accepted this, but my heart was impatient. I had an agenda that breast surgery was not part of. Many years previously we as a family had hosted, more than once, a visiting French student. He had come to us because the organisation bringing him to England wanted 'a sympathetic household' for a teenager who was profoundly deaf. At the time, we were mystified as to why that should be a definition of our home! From the first, however, it was we who were privileged. Our visitor was delightful. He lip-read English or French with equal ease, fitted in well with our son, teased our daughter 'big brother' fashion (he was considerably older than both of them and part of a big family) and we quickly grew to love him – and not just him, but, when we subsequently met them, the entire family. The summer that I had my surgery, he was to be married. We had promised, the previous July, that we would be there. I wasn't about to let my disease get in the way if I could help it…

After the surgery, I had two drains and in excess of twenty staples in my chest. The movement in my left arm was severely limited. It is necessary after lymphectomy to work hard at specific physiotherapy exercises to regain the movement in the upper arm and shoulder. Some people never make a full recovery. I felt that I really must, if only for the pleasure of playing my guitar! After about three days, the drains were removed. Now it was possible to start exercising in earnest, and Xiao Yan and I paced each other and monitored each other's progress. That way we both did well. I was determined to be sufficiently recovered to attend that wedding in France, which was to take place ten days after my surgery and one day before I was due to have my staples removed. My surgeon was most encouraging and didn't seem to perceive any problem with that.

Meanwhile, the bed that had been taken by the paralysed lady the night after my surgery had a new occupant; a lovely lady whom I will call Julie. Julie was older than me, and shared with me the fact that she saw little point in caring for, or about, anyone other than her immediate family. Though her children were quite grown up, it became apparent that she was still a very good and caring mother. What troubled me was that she seemed to care very little about herself. She said that she had no faith and saw no higher purpose. Despite these things, I really enjoyed talking to her, for she had many entertaining and likeable qualities. I told her as much, complimenting her upon the things that were so obviously heart-warming about her, and she bristled: 'Why are you being nice to me? Do you want something?' I told her, yes, I wanted her to feel good about herself – her many positive attributes. Within a day or two she was gone and I have not seen her since, but as she left she admonished me sternly to, 'Stay the way you are.' I would like to think that God used our conversations to show her just a little of her own real value as a unique and special person. At any rate, I was privileged to have met and talked to her and I felt that I had seen her defensive shell begin to melt…Who knows what might lie beneath?

After five days I was discharged. I went home and faithfully did my prescribed exercises. I had to revisit the ward to have some swelling examined. It was caused by fluid that was tracking down my ribcage; lymphatic fluid was travelling down my back under the skin and pooling above my waist, but no treatment was needed and it eventually dispersed. I went to France for the wedding, complete with my staples.

Madness it was. We got up at four that morning and arrived home at one the next, and I really paid for it the day after but

I wouldn't have missed it for the world. There was a civil ceremony followed by a beautiful church wedding and I loved the hymns, one of which was Patrick Richard's lovely song 'Tout un chemin pour te chercher'. It speaks so eloquently of wanting to learn to love better – to give everything to God – verse one very specifically handing over all aspects, joyful or sorrowful, of the singer's life, thanking God for all that He has given and responding with a 'yes' to Him in all circumstances… all!

At the time, I found those words very powerful. Anything that God allowed to happen to me He would ultimately use for my good. If I trusted in that, I had no choice but to say my own 'yes' and try to mean it!

It was a lovely, lovely wedding and a beautiful day amongst caring friends who assured me my prognosis was good, urged us to stay on, but wished us well when it became clear we had made up our minds to leave, and warmly promised to see us in early September.

On the way back to the ferry, as my husband and myself and our two children sat in the car, there was time for both reflection and conversation, which quickly became heated. My children were both angry. Both had independently reached the conclusion that I had cancer. Both felt that we, as parents, had not been entirely honest with them; had not, in fact, treated them as the young adults that they had become. Our son felt that we sometimes chided him for not being sufficiently helpful and sympathetic, yet we had played down my sickness to the extent that it seemed 'no big deal', so what need was there for a big effort at help or sympathy? Our daughter had gone to the mother of her closest friend and asked, 'Do you think it sounds like cancer?' I felt awful. I had taken advice from the consultant and from the breast care nurses about what to say, and then I had tried to do my best without being unduly alarming. Now I felt that I had failed. My husband and I both felt the anger and resentment in our children and listened to what they had to say. Next time, we promised, we would try to treat them as responsible adults and tell them the whole truth.

'Next time' was not long in coming. I had the staples removed from my wound shortly after returning from France, but the breast was still very painful and the wound not entirely healed. The involved breast was now about one quarter to one third smaller than the other one, but I felt I could live with that; lots of women don't 'match' so why should I worry?... But I wasn't healing as quickly as I had hoped and I was concerned about the approaching histology report...

The histology report comes in two weeks after the surgery, and until it does, you do not really know what you are dealing with. I went with Martin, my husband, to the clinic, and was seen by appointment. Just as my surgeon was about to start speaking to me, the breast care nurse came in, obviously by appointment. At the time, I said to her, 'If you're here, it's not good news.' I've since learned that I was in error; women receiving good (as many do) or bad news in such emotionally charged circumstances may well misunderstand and have need of another friendly pair of ears attached to someone with sympathy and medical understanding; such is the breast care nurse.

The report was not all that we had hoped for. Though the excision had been wide, it had not had, as was planned, a nice wide area of uninvolved tissue around it. Instead, the histology showed, I had widespread ductal carcinoma – there was a lot of early cancer left in my breast. More worrying still, of the fifteen lymph nodes that had been taken from under my left arm (causing me to go through a painful exercise regime every day in order to regain full movement) five were involved – the cancer had spread from my breast tissue to my lymph system.

This was not what we had wanted to hear. I found it very difficult to take on board in some ways. After all, I had found the cancer myself, after the doctor had given me a clean bill of health, so I had assumed I had found it early. The whole point had been to avoid walking in my mother's footsteps and now I felt I was doing just that. Crazy, really. We are all unique and each one of us has our own, special journey. Even the type of cancer was completely different and unrelated in any way to my mother's. The report showed a grade three cancer. That's the type you don't want. They come as grade one, two, or three, three being the most invasive. Grade one would have done me fine! Not only that, but the fact that it had spread to the lymph nodes was not good news; we were supposed to have caught it...

It was explained to us that I would have to have a mastectomy... We'd gone for the lump initially, now we'd have to go for the breast. The primary tumour had been 1.7 centimetres, but the cancerous area of the breast was much larger... And after the mastectomy, I would have to have chemotherapy because the cancer had spread to my lymph nodes... We were taken to a side room and counselled, given time to adjust and ask questions. Everything had a slightly unreal quality and yet an inevitability about it.

We talked about so many things in that little room. I was shown various breast prostheses and I had real concern, because I remembered that my mother, dead these eighteen years, had had terrible problems, once she had a prosthetic breast, in trying to get her rather large breasts to hang level. At one point, my father had opened up a foam prosthesis and put a weight into it for her. My mother had been a size 38DD. I was a size 34G or H. This meant I had a smaller ribcage, but bigger breasts. How would I cope and what would I look like with just one…? I felt that I would look ludicrous. Moreover, in these enlightened times, it is usual to offer women instant reconstruction, should they wish it, or, if they prefer to defer it, reconstruction at a later date, which many surgeons feel is the wiser option. Reconstruction sounds like a great idea. Instant reconstruction sounds even better. Who wouldn't want to wake up with a new breast in place of the one they had lost? But there's a catch…or there was in my case, because there was no way that I could have a reconstruction that came anywhere near to matching the size of my remaining breast. If I had opted for reconstruction, a smaller breast would have been built in place of the one I had lost. I would then have been committed to having surgery to reduce the remaining breast to a similar size. I remember being very concerned about this prospect at the time for very personal reasons: bluntly, I would be likely to lose all nipple sensitivity in the right breast when it was reduced and this seemed a big deal to me, as I was about to lose the left breast altogether. What kind of a sexual being could I be in the future, I wondered?

I was counselled, I think wisely, that 'in my case' instant reconstruction would not be a good idea. Had I opted for it, I would have had to wait longer for surgery and I would have had to wear a partial prosthesis over the reconstructed breast until the chemotherapy was completed, because surgery to the other breast would not be possible until the chemo was finished. Persons on chemo have compromised immunity and poor rates of healing. Also, the original wound had not yet healed, and I wanted to get on with the next surgery as soon as possible. It seemed crazy to heal up and then have to be cut in the same area all over again, repeating the process, but there are waiting lists, and many women go through the shattering experience of breast cancer, and in fact there were, as it turned out, four weeks between my surgeries.

The wait was not easy. Meanwhile, there were other issues to address. I was counselled about chemotherapy. Broadly, there were two types on offer, and the oncologist, whom I would meet on the day that the histology report from the mastectomy came in, would decide on the kind that was appropriate for me. The decision would be based on all the evidence relating to my specific condition, and would be designed to give the best outcome for me. One kind of chemotherapy, I was informed, would be administered fortnightly for six months. It would not result in total hair loss, though the hair would thin. The other, more aggressive, regime would be administered perhaps monthly, usually for four months, and would result in total hair loss, but would be over sooner. (I think I may have been a little confused when I received this information. I later learned that this chemotherapy is usually six cycles of three weeks each and it may be that I was told this at this time and misunderstood – but I feel it is important to report what I understood at the time, because this whole experience was a process and a learning curve.) There was a possibility that I would need some radiotherapy as well.

So, I would lose my breast, and the nurses who would help me to find an appropriate prosthesis had to admit that they could not actually remember if they had ever fitted anyone like me before…and I may well lose my hair as well…and now we were warned about something else, too.

In one of life's ironic twists, we discovered that I was actually more likely to conceive now than I had been before, because I was on Tamoxifen. Sometimes, Tamoxifen is used to help treat some forms of sub-fertility. Apparently, patients on chemotherapy can also still conceive. To do so would result in instant tragedy, we were told at this time. (Later, I discovered that others hold a different view). The woman, we were told, would immediately be offered an abortion because there was no possibility of a positive outcome. A developing baby would be likely to be terribly harmed by chemotherapy drugs, and the mother would be dreadfully harmed by the hormones, surging around her body during pregnancy, on which her cancer depended. It may well progress out of control...

Abortion would be unthinkable to us; we had never even used contraception, and now they were telling us that we must not risk pregnancy for the duration of the treatment or for about two years afterwards... Were we to lose the comfort of our loving relationship as well as my hair and my breast? It didn't bear thinking about... Yet we had to think, and to agonise...

What I have since learned, but was not told at this time, is that there has been some research reported from America which suggests that, if a woman conceives on chemotherapy, one of two things will happen. Either the baby will spontaneously abort, or the pregnancy will proceed successfully to term without harm to the developing child. Indeed, some mothers, properly cared for, have experienced very positive outcomes. However, since the mother in question is likely to have a cancer which will feed on the hormones present in her body in greater quantities during pregnancy, any possibility of pregnancy in such a person has to be considered dangerous and undesirable and as such to be avoided.

On a seemingly trivial and much more practical level, we were advised that, should I need a wig, we would be told where to go for the best options for me. The hospital provides its own service, but can also advise on other outlets outside, and the cost is always roughly the same, about £70.00 at the time of writing. Beside the life and death considerations relating to our love life, we were considering the cost of fake hair! The feeling of unreality deepened…

When we left the hospital that day, we were both somewhat in shock. We had accepted that, for me, there would be no instant reconstruction. Quite apart from the considerations of size, there was the problem of a possible adverse allergic reaction. I have many known allergies; what if I was to have an allergic reaction to the silicon bag filled with saline that would be used in such a reconstruction? The likely result would be further surgery to remove the implant…

Back home, I did as I had promised I would do: I told my children the whole truth about the content of the histology report and the path forward from that. Our son was at home. He was extremely shaken by the news and at first did not fully understand it. It was my fault; I had not realised that he did not know that 'mastectomy' meant removal of the breast. How should he know? It was not an everyday term and was hardly relevant to an intelligent and active young man in his teens. I was so used to such terms by now that I had not properly explained. It was several days before we were able to talk freely and I explained this to him. Also, in his mind, chemotherapy was something given to those beyond all other help. I did explain that I was to receive preventive chemotherapy, intended to mop up any stray cancer cells that may exist, and that this was rather different, but sometimes there is an impression already in place that might be hard to shift, however good the explanation.

Our daughter was away from home at university so I had to tell her on the phone. She wept. She wept a lot. I was not able to hug her. I was left feeling that, even though this time I had done exactly what my children said they wanted, I had somehow got it wrong again. Now I feel that such a situation is in some ways inevitable; I don't believe there is a right way to handle this scenario for which there are no rehearsals. We are all simply human and the only thing one can do in such circumstances is to do the best you can and leave the rest to God. I have also learned that, when a child appears to direct extreme anger at the parent in such a situation, it is the cancer they really want to target. There is just no way that they can do so.

As I have said, the wait for the mastectomy was hard. The hospital staff were doing all they could to get me in as soon as possible. Meanwhile, I had a left breast which, though considerably smaller than the right now, was large, pendulous, improperly healed and painful, and even if further healing did take place, I would only be cut again. In my ignorance, I had thought that much of my discomfort would be alleviated once the staples were removed, but the wound, a long one, had continued to be painful and to weep. I applied clean handkerchiefs and later gauze that the hospital supplied, but it all seemed so futile when the breast was going anyway. When I could, I went to work and tried to think of something else. I seldom succeeded.

During this period I went over the details of my histology report with the breast care nurse, using the telephone contact number I had used so many times before. It was helpful because she assured me that the fact that only five of my fifteen lymph nodes were involved (cancerous) was positive news. I eventually also learned that my tumour was heavily dependent on progestogen and weakly dependent on oestrogen (both natural hormones produced in the body). I would be medicated to lower the circulating levels of such hormones via the Tamoxifen.

Martin and I prayerfully sought spiritual advice, to help us to make decisions about our personal lives, from trusted sources of counsel. We were terribly concerned at the information we had been given about the impossibility of any positive outcome, should I become pregnant. It is not perhaps appropriate to record here exactly what we decided, since for every couple that finds itself upon that road, there may be a different but equally appropriate route to walk. Suffice it to say that we took the advice of two clergymen we trusted, and both independently gave very similar counsel. I am indebted to them for their warmth and understanding at a time when I felt so very vulnerable and so much at sea in so many ways. I will say, however, that both advisers told us, amongst other things, that they did not feel that abstinence from our loving sexual relationship would be appropriate; we needed each other and our closeness if we were to cope. I believe this was very sound advice.

One thing that has always given me tremendous pleasure is my role in the music ministry. There had been a hole in my life, and when God found me a place in the music ministry, He filled that hole. I could never have been a professional musician; I simply don't have the talent. But by the grace of God, there is a lot of music in me, and I love having the opportunity to let it out in His service. Accordingly, though much of my life was now on hold, I sought to continue to play and sing. One regular fixture in the band's music calendar was a fortnightly visit to a Christian healing prayer group (though the prayer group was based in a Roman Catholic parish, all were welcome) in the London area. The congregation was usually up to about sixty people and we were well known there. These good people had been very supportive with their prayer and sent a wonderful card full of warm wishes. Now the leader asked me to address a meeting and tell them in person what was happening to me.

I shared with them a brief account of the treatment I had still to receive. I also shared with them my belief that God would not permit something as devastating as this to happen to me unless He intended to bring great blessings out of it for me and those close to me. This was a belief I held very strongly and with good reason.

On Friday nights, we played at a smaller local prayer group made up of mixed Christian denominations. Sometimes, during quiet times in the course of the meetings, I was blessed with mental pictures which deepened my spiritual understanding. Around the time when my journey with cancer was beginning, I had seen such a picture; one that at first I did not understand. I saw a shell – a pretty, curly one with mother of pearl inside it, some grains of sand beside the shell, and some pearls beside the grains of sand. At the time, I had not understood the significance of the images, thinking they maybe had to do with the diversity of God's creation, but as I was driving home after the meeting I had to stop at traffic lights and suddenly, in that enforced pause, I knew exactly what it meant, and knew it so clearly. It all just popped into my head in that instant. The shell represented my breast. The grains of sand represented the calcium deposits within it which had been the means of initial diagnosis, and the pearls represented the good things that God was going to bring out of this experience for me and mine. Subsequently, I shared this interpretation with the members of the Friday prayer group and one dear friend there bought me a pearl (the first of many that came to me following this revelation) while she was holidaying in the Balearics. I wore it every day for a long while, to remind me of the good that would come…

Thus it was that I felt confident to tell the London prayer group congregation to watch this space for good things! Having brought them up to date on my progress, I returned to my seat. At the break time in the middle of the proceedings, a lady who is a regular there came to speak to me. I truly think that God wanted us to have our conversation. She told me about a recently published book. It wasn't a Christian book, it was a book written by someone who had herself journeyed through breast cancer and beaten it. It was called 'Your Life In Your Hands', she said, and she also told me the name of the author, but at the time there was so much going on around me that I didn't note this. I believe that God wanted me to know about this book because its content was one of the tools He was going to use to help me. God bless the good lady who drew my attention to it!

On the telephone the next day, I mentioned the book to my father. He, thoughtful man that he is, telephoned a bookshop in my area, one that we know has a great postal service, and they were able to tell him who the author was – Professor Jane Plant – and to post me a copy at his expense. The book made astonishing reading in many ways and, in a way that is rare among 'health' books, could substantiate its claims with copious reference notes, referring to sound sources. I found it immeasurably helpful. One of my local prayer group friends told me, 'I believe you were meant to find and read that book.' I believe so too. On the strength of its arguments, I immediately gave up eating or drinking any form of dairy produce, largely substituting soya. I still believe this to have been a crucial move. I was also grateful because here was something which I could do and which, it appeared from the evidence, might really help me to fight the disease.

Returning to hospital, initially I was placed in a single side ward, but a nurse who remembered me from my previous visit said, 'You're a social person. You'll be better with others. Come with me.' Thanks to her, I ended up in the bed next to the one I had occupied on my previous visit. I almost felt at home, partly because of where I was and partly because so many of the staff remembered me and they were so very kind and warm in their approach. My surgery would take place the next day. After the seemingly interminable wait for a bed, everything was now moving fast, and I was grateful.

I awoke many times during that night. A lady had been admitted to the bed next to mine, barely conscious and in constant pain. She was not able to stop herself from crying out, neither was she capable of understanding that in order to call the nurse she must press the orange call button. She would simply call, 'Nurse! Nurse!' but the nursing station was halfway down the main ward corridor and we were in a side bay at the beginning of it. There was no way that the nurse could hear her call. Only the other three women in the bay could hear her, and throughout the night we took turns in pressing our own call buttons to alert the nurses to her plight. When lucid, she would apologise to us and of course we told her not to worry. We knew that she couldn't help herself...but by about two in the morning I felt desperate and ashamed, because I could bear the disturbances no longer and they seemed to be coming about every ten minutes. I would just be drifting into a restless sleep when I would be jolted out again by her piercing or pained cries. I did not want to upset her or to wake the others but I just could not cope. I stumbled out onto the corridor where I could not be heard and I sobbed. I was having a hard time living with the thought of what was to be done to me next day, and listening to the agony of this poor woman and being powerless to alleviate it was just too much. The nurses had told her that she had had all the pain killers they could administer; what could *I* then do? And yet she cried out still.

It was cold on the corridor and I was so tired, yet sleep was far from me. The night nurse came and found me. She took me to the nurses' station and made me a drink with my soya milk (they had from the start been totally accommodating about my desire to be on a non-dairy diet). Then we talked for a long time about breast cancer, and my mum and *her* mum (see how God provides the person who knows!) and advances in treatment and about why I was *not* just following in my mother's footsteps. She was so kind and so understanding and it helped. She also explained to me that the lady who was in so much pain would definitely get well, and that some of the time when, semi-conscious, she cried out, it was for the comfort of hearing a human voice reply, in order to help her to orientate herself, as she felt lost in her strange surroundings. Who, then, could withhold such reassurance? I returned to bed and finally slept, comforted in myself and with a better understanding of my current neighbour.

Morning came and I was first on the list. Last time I had gone to theatre I had been in comparatively good spirits. The staff had taken their time over administering the anaesthetic and there had been much good-natured banter, but now it was different. I had wept at work a few days before. It had suddenly seemed so unreasonable that they were going to cut my breast off. How could I ever look right again? Now, faced with the imminence of the operation, I was weeping again. The nurses were great. Was I concerned that my husband wouldn't fancy me? They were very anxious to reassure me that he still would – but I knew that. What concerned me was that *I* wouldn't fancy me! I didn't know how I was going to live with the results of this day's work. But, they reminded me, it was a life saving operation and I really didn't have a choice…and I didn't, because whatever

I felt about the road ahead, I had a loving husband and two wonderful children and I owed it to them to do everything I could to try to get well... Yet I was weeping and weeping and it seemed I could not stop. Once again, I was vulnerable, stripped, without my jewellery, my badges of identity, my toe-nail polish. Once again, it was just the Lord and me. I knew His care for me was just as great this time, but the enormity of it all was overwhelming...and I just couldn't stop crying.

My close friend Gemma is a midwife. She works in the same hospital where my surgery took place. She had promised to visit me before reporting to her ward on the day of my surgery. That would have been at about a quarter past seven in the morning, but she had not appeared, and now they were wheeling me down to the lifts, the tears streaming down my face...and there she was! As we reached the lifts, she walked through the doors from the stairs, and characteristically threw herself into my arms. She is tiny and neatly built, and consequently, once she embraced me, was more or less in the bed with me, but the other staff didn't seem to mind and wheeled us both down to theatre regardless, as she prayed over me and comforted me.

At the theatre doors we said goodbye, and I, still weeping uncontrollably, was wheeled in. It was all so different this time. There was no banter. No one playfully propositioned me. Does anyone, I wondered, *want* to proposition a woman who will soon have only one breast, even in fun? And what of a one-breasted woman who may soon be bald as well? The tears just kept coming, and the anaesthetists worked fast. They were even a little rough in their speed, almost, it seemed, forcing syringes of fluid into the canula in the back of my hand, so that they hurt, stinging as they went in, but they would work speedily and speed was of the essence...They knew that. They were gifting me with sleep to put a temporary end to the wailing misery. 'Nothing we can say,' they told me, 'will make you feel better, so...' and I drifted out of consciousness.

This time, when I awoke, I was pain-free. I had two lines in my arm. One was a drip to ensure that I did not become dehydrated; the other was an apparatus to enable me to deliver morphine by pressing a button, to obtain pain relief at need. I also, once again, had two drains in my chest... in the flat side... At least, this time, when my husband and son visited, I was able to talk with them, drifting in and out of drowsiness. I was not hurting, physically, and that was a great blessing.

From the time of my first diagnosis, I had been overwhelmed by people's kindness. I had a wonderful family and many good friends, I knew, but colleagues, members of the churches I attended, people who lived in our street, relatives who usually contacted us only annually at Christmas – the list went on and on – all of these people sent me their warm thoughts and good wishes. Very many of them came to visit me and many brought thoughtful gifts. One brought me three horse chestnuts ('conkers' as we call them), to remind me that God spells 'conquers' in a more meaningful way! I will never be able to explain to these people the true value of their unstinting support. I had done nothing to deserve it and I felt unworthy, but the waves of warmth, the cards, the flowers and the visitors just kept coming. I knew the prayers were just as constant. Friends connected with the music ministry were particularly faithful. They will never know how much I valued those visits, how much I love them for the strength they brought to me then. People often feel powerless, faced with a friend or a family member who has cancer. They think, 'What can *I* do?' In fact, it is the *being there* that matters; their very presence is what is needed, and in their simple words and visits is the strength that the sick person draws upon.

Morphine as a pain killer is a great blessing, but morphine is also a 'brain-killer' because it confuses your perception and sense of reality. For the day and a half during which I pressed that button and sent the welcome relief surging into my arm, my recollection of what really took place is coloured by distortions caused by the drug. However, there are some things that were terribly frightening at the time that I remember clearly...

I had a very clear recollection of what the surgeon had said he would do. I trusted him completely. I still do. He is a marvellous and dedicated man who takes very great care of his patients and very great pride in his work. He had told me that he would take away all of my left breast and any remaining lymph nodes. I had known that there was a kind of mastectomy called a 'radical mastectomy' in which the underlying chest muscles were also taken. The breast care nurse told me that this kind of surgery would **not** be done; indeed it was rarely done nowadays. 'You would be very disfigured,' she had said. Yet, when I looked in the mirror, I was not just flat. The area under my collar bone was concave, but only on the left side. I did not understand what this could mean. The incision itself was covered by a dressing, with a drain tube anchored at either end.

I was further puzzled because, by the lack of discomfort in that area, I knew that the surgeon had *not* removed any remaining lymph nodes from my armpit. Did this mean he had forgotten? Would I have to go back into theatre and be opened up again? One of the house doctors called to try to answer my question. He said that he had missed the first part of the operation, but he was sure that the surgeon must have done everything that was necessary. I have to say that at the time I did not find this entirely reassuring. Later, however, the surgeon himself, my consultant, came by. It was after hours. He had been told of my anxiety and had dropped by to reassure me. At the lumpectomy, he said, he had removed fifteen lymph nodes, of which five were involved, that is to say invaded by cancer. Not many people have more nodes in the axilla, he explained, but, had he seen more, he would have removed them. In the event, the reason he had not done any further work under my arm was because there had been no more work to do. Everything appeared cleared and disease free. As regards the apparent hollowness of my chest, he explained that, statistically, a surgeon leaves behind between five and fifteen percent of breast tissue when performing a mastectomy. He himself, he explained, tried very hard to leave as little as possible. He removed the breast and all associated fat. He said that the hollow area would gradually build up again over the next year. I had no need to be concerned. Grateful for this man's kindness and reassured by his out of hours visit, I slept.

Next day, I was visited by the same house doctor who had seen me on the day of my surgery. He examined my wound and told me, as the surgeon had before him, that they would need to keep an eye on it. This had somehow not seemed so fearful when the surgeon had said it, but perhaps I had not had so much morphine then… I understood from the surgeon that 'in my case' (would I ever stop hearing those three words?) it had been necessary to close a larger wound than was usual, and this meant that the skin (previously the underside of my breast) which had been used for the closure of the wound was not necessarily adequately supplied with blood for good healing. Consequently, one area of the 'seam' looked very dark and bruised and would need to be monitored…

The words 'Do not be afraid' occur, I am told, three hundred and sixty five times in the Bible – once for each day of the year –

but I was very raw and very vulnerable and maybe that explains a great deal about what happened next…

…Now the house doctor was looking at this same dark area and telling his team the same thing about monitoring, but he added some words that were instantly alarming to me; 'This can be a problem.' My antennae were up! 'What do you mean?' I asked him. 'Well,' he responded, 'if it doesn't heal, it can be a problem.' By now, I was thoroughly alarmed. Was he telling me that I had a hole in my chest that would not heal? What would they do? I asked him and he replied that they would keep an eye on it. I did not find this particularly reassuring. What kind of problem was he talking about I asked him? Did he mean MRSA or perhaps gangrene? What *did* he mean when he said so mysteriously that it 'could be a problem' and yet offered no further information, no solution? This was a huge wound on my chest we were talking about, and it was not even the usual almost straight line that most mastectomy patients have. *In my case* (those words again), it had been necessary to make a curved incision in an arc from my sternum to my armpit. There were, in fact, forty-two staples in my chest. I waited for him to explain what would be done to solve the problem, should it occur, but he told the team that I was clearly becoming distressed (too right, I was!) and that I had been distressed the day before when I was taken to theatre, and he thought they should move on! The whole team left, leaving the curtains drawn around my bed, since I was clearly so upset. This still seems to me to have been a curious response to my circumstances; perhaps it was caused by a lack of empathy? Who can tell?

Now I was *really* alarmed. What on earth had the man meant? Remember, I could not think clearly because of my morphine-fuddled brain and I felt so scared at the prospect of a problem with no solution. Once again, I was sobbing. The nurse came to comfort me and said that, as far as she could see, my wound was doing fine. She felt that I needed to talk to someone and tried to contact the breast care nurses, without success. She asked me if she could contact my husband. Perhaps his presence would reassure me.

Eventually, they called Martin. They told him that his wife had seen the doctor and was upset, so could he possibly visit and comfort her? Consequently, the poor man was stuck in London traffic enduring mind games about what terrible prognosis the doctor could possibly have disclosed. He rang my midwife friend, who was at home off duty, and asked if she was in a position to get to me. She came within a very short time to the ward. She listened to my account of the morning's visit and expressed concern. She was sure that there wasn't really a problem in terms of my eventual health, more a problem in terms of communication. She helped me to have a wash, escorted me to the toilet (not easy when you are trailing four tubes and attached to a drip stand) and stayed with me until Martin came. Thankful for such support, I became calmer.

Later that day one of the senior lady doctors on the team visited me. Strictly speaking, she was not my doctor, but she sat down beside me and explained, first of all, about the lymph nodes – that any remaining lymph nodes that I had in that area would be up in my neck. There they would be close to many delicate structures which could easily be harmed if any attempt was made to dissect them out. There was no reason, she said, to believe that any such nodes were diseased, but even if there had been, an alternative method of treating them, such as radiotherapy, would have been chosen because of the dangers of surgery. She also reinforced for me the rightness of my decision not to go for any kind of instant reconstruction 'in my case', explaining in detail what would have to happen to the right breast to make it match a reconstructed left one. She drew diagrams to explain clearly to me this obviously quite major surgery…What, I wondered, would I ultimately wish to do? Then she explained about the 'problem' with the wound. I did not need to be alarmed, she said. If the skin that was causing the concern did in fact have an inadequate blood supply, it would effectively die back, but then either the wound would be resectioned with good skin at the closure point *or* treated with special dressings to encourage the growth of new skin, like a wound caused by a burn, *or* a skin graft could be used to heal it. There were lots of possibilities. Then why, I asked, hadn't the other doctor told me these things? Why had he allowed me to become so very frightened?

Now, on reflection, I believe it was a combination of factors that put me into such a state of fear that day. For sure, the morphine didn't help the clarity of my thinking, but also, English was not the first language of the house doctor and maybe the stress of my panic made it hard for him to find the right words. He was young; perhaps he was also relatively inexperienced. Possibly, the more upset I became, the more uncomfortable he felt and the less able he was to search for the words he wanted to use for reassurance. Probably he had in fact decided to cut his losses and leave before I became still further disturbed and the situation worsened. At any rate, he came back after hours to see me, in the calm of the evening, and when I said, 'You frightened me,' he said, 'I told you we'd keep an eye on it.' I guess the whole episode *was* one of miscommunication.

Seeing the plate of food in front of me, he asked if I was enjoying my dinner. There were a few potatoes and some broccoli florets posing as islands in an absolute sea of brown minced meat. They had been very good about supplying non-dairy food, but I hadn't expected them to grind up the cow and try to feed it to me! Now that they had, I couldn't eat it. At least the two of us had a laugh about that.

The lady doctor's visit that afternoon had done me a great deal of good. She had been so patient, had explained so clearly, drawing little diagrams as necessary, and had treated my concerns seriously, ensuring that I understood. I have met her many times since and never found her manner any different. Thank God for her empathy; this is as healing to her patients as her medical skills.

One event that does deserve a mention, which arose partly as a result of all the concern about my wound and how it would heal, revealed to me just how uncertain were my emotional responses at this stage of my treatment. I had bravely allowed my daughter to see the site of the latest surgery when she asked, drains and all (though the incision site itself was covered by a large sticking plaster dressing). I had tried to look down and see my new self and to accept it whenever anyone else was examining me. I thought I was pretty together on that score, yet on one of the evenings shortly after the surgery I took myself to the bathroom for a wash and, when I undressed, I fell apart completely.

I had been wearing a button-through night-shirt, and on reaching the basin I ripped open the buttons…The dressing over the wound had completely fallen away, having been loosened by all the medical staff that had previously pulled it to one side to inspect the wound. It was now hanging by a small strip of sticky tape on one side – and I was staring at myself in a long mirror with nothing to hide the full devastation of what had happened to my body.

There on the right was a very full and obvious breast. On the left there was a dark blood-coloured gash, purple in parts, with metal staples (forty-two, as I have already said) along its length.

The gash stretched from the centre of my chest to my armpit, in an upward curve. At each end of it there was a drain tube curling away, red from the blood it was carrying. At that time it was just too much to be confronted with my true reflection in this way. I simply could not cope. Drawing my night-shirt back around me and abandoning my toiletries in the bathroom, I dashed out onto the corridor. I don't think I knew where I was going, but I headed towards the nurses' station.

Seeing my distress, the sister asked what had happened. Gently, she established that the bald confrontation with the actual state of my body under the dressings had been a great shock. I was led into the treatment room and my wound was re-dressed, then I went once more to wash, this time seeing only white dressing strips between the drain tubes when I caught myself in the mirror. Many things we can cope with, in due time, but there are occasions when time is the very thing we need, in order to be able to adjust – 'To everything there is a season'.

Following this incident, I was to be amazed once more at how God uses us, even when we are at our very weakest. There was a lady in our ward whom I shall call Toni. In the dark of the late evening, as we were settling down for the night, Toni shared a pressing anxiety she had with the rest of us. A friend had told her that at least part of the reason for the sickness she was suffering was her inability to forgive someone who had done her a great wrong – that carrying that anger and lack of forgiveness inside her had helped to make her so sick. It doesn't matter whether this could be true or not – what matters is that Toni believed it, and the whole idea troubled her greatly. Personally, I feel that it is very possible that carrying repressed hurt can make a person sick; I have also experienced the liberating power of forgiveness. Toni was in difficulties because she accepted what she had been told, and for her it was now necessary to do something about it. She wanted to find a way to forgive the person who had hurt her but that person, an adult male family member who had sexually abused her as a child, had since died, and so was beyond her reach. Moreover, Toni was still hurting. The injustice stung her and she did not know how she could let go of the hurt…

I listened very carefully to what she had to say, as did the others in the ward, and between us, two of us hatched a suggestion, not of ourselves, I was convinced, but with prompting from the Lord, who had at so many times shown Himself present in this whole scenario.

There must have been a time, we said, when this relative was just an innocent little boy, playing with friends in the garden. Could she, perhaps, imagine herself visiting him then and there? As a child, he could pose no threat to her and it would be safe for her to love him and to tell him of her forgiveness. Perhaps this way, she could put down her burden of sorrow?

Eventually, we all slept. By the time I awoke next morning, Toni was absolutely radiant. During the dark of the night, she had made a mental pilgrimage to a back garden in this man's childhood. She had met with him in his innocence and frailty and she had told him that she forgave him for the weaknesses of his later life that had caused her so much pain. By the grace of God, she was at last free of this huge burden. Her face and her manner were transformed. I marvel at the way God works. It was very humbling to have been present; such a privilege and such a blessing to have met Toni, seen the beautiful person that she was, and to have shared this special moment in her life.

On yet another occasion while I was in that ward, I felt really strongly the presence of God's grace. A friend, Michael, from the Friday prayer group had felt moved to send me a particular text just before I went into the hospital. To be honest, at the time I pondered over it, wondering why he was so sure it would be relevant to what was about to happen. I have to say that, in those particular circumstances, it seemed a really odd choice to me and I could see no connection whatsoever...

One night, I got talking to Mabel, an elderly lady in the ward. As people do at times like these, she was talking about how faith sustained her, but, she shared with me, she had felt great sorrow over her father. I asked why, and she explained that her father had not been a man of faith; he had seemed indifferent to such things. However, one night, some time after the death of her mother, Mabel had passed her father's bedroom door and seen him on his knees in prayer. I said that was great, but she said yes, but it troubled her...all the time that he had lost...coming to the Lord so late in his life... And at that point, I understood, and I reached for the text which had seemed so irrelevant and read it to her... 'I will repay the years the locusts have eaten...' it ran. At that moment I experienced a sense of absolute awe at God's providence and timing!

On the third day after the mastectomy, I was allowed home. I'm not sure that I was really ready to go; the nursing staff had said that I could stay if I wished, but I think you somehow feel that if they think you're ready to go, then go you should. Certainly, I was in many ways frail, perhaps particularly emotionally. I rang my husband and it was immediately obvious that my call had thrown him into confusion. The reason, as I later found out, was that some friends had been working in the garden, trying to ensure that a small water feature that some of them had given to me for my birthday was up and running by the time I came home – and no one had expected me home so soon! I had other issues on my mind...

From the first, once I had known I would need a mastectomy, I had been concerned about how I would look. The breast care nurses had assured me that, after the surgery, someone would see me on the ward and would make sure that the 'comfy' that I would be given initially (a cotton breast form filled with soft padding, to wear in place of my missing breast) would be sufficiently substantial to match the other one, if necessary adding to the stuffing inside it to achieve a good balance. In the event, due to build up of numbers on the patient waiting list, my surgery had taken place on an added day. This meant I hadn't slotted into the normal weekly programme where certain things tend to happen on certain half-days. Now I was being discharged before I had seen anyone from the breast care team on the ward.

A friend who had had a mastectomy had told me all about the catalogues she was given, showing various prostheses and suitable underwear, lingerie and swimwear. I had seen nothing of the sort whilst in hospital, though I had responded to some small advertisements and ordered catalogues which had been delivered to my home. I had also ordered two new sports bras which were of a substantial camisole type and which I hoped would stay in place better than some, as I tried to get to grips with my new self. So here I was, preparing to go home, and where was the expected support? It was nobody's fault, but I had been led to believe that it would be there for me and it appeared that it was not.

In the event, one of the nurses came to my rescue. They were a wonderful team, those nurses, because they understood the issues so well and could almost second-guess the minds of their charges. Also, they did not lose patience with us. They would cover the same ground again and again as necessary to help an individual understand or come to terms with something, and their good humour never failed, even under stress. They were living a God-given vocation and a true ministry.

On this occasion, the nurse suggested that I come down to the treatment room with my bra. In this room there was a good mirror. She and I would stand together in front of this and would do whatever it took to get it right. It would be O.K., she promised me, and so, in fact it was. A 'comfy' designed for a lady with a much larger bra size than my own 34, and who might require a DD cup size, turned out to fit the bill very well. I stuffed it into the empty side of my bra, we played a bit with the straps to get things level (polyester just doesn't have the weight that a breast has) and I was away! Once dressed, it was amazing how normal I looked. In fact, I looked good. I had lost a little weight and appeared trim and fit. However, I still had a long way to go…inside.

I was home! The water feature was running in the garden, I was resting in a chair; there were cards and good wishes all around me and the surgery was over, so I should have been feeling good. Yet there were issues. There would be another histology report, following this surgery, and I hadn't enjoyed receiving the last one. Also, I knew already that I would have to receive chemotherapy, once I had fully healed from the surgery. And, once again, there were the arm exercises… At least these were a little less painful because, during the most recent surgery, the surgeon had released some tissues that had been restrictively tight following my earlier operation and I now had much greater mobility. I *would*, I felt, regain the full range of arm movement on that side. (And I surely have! Persistence pays off.)

Persons who have had their lymph nodes removed do not have the same ability to fight infection in the affected part of their body as the remainder of the population has. Consequently, ladies like me are issued with a laminated card to carry in our handbags. This card states that blood pressure readings and blood tests may not be conducted on the affected side. We are counselled to wear gloves for domestic work and gardening and to keep disinfectant and antiseptic handy. Cuts must be promptly dealt with, cleaned and disinfected, and any heating up of the area following an injury must be viewed with concern. In such an event, medical advice must be sought in case there *is* an infection. We are told that we must be responsible for looking after ourselves, taking proper care of the affected arm. This can seem like yet another limitation in a lifestyle already prematurely restricted. It is not much to worry about while you sit in a chair and convalesce, but who wants to do that for ever?

Prior to my illness I had been a keen gardener, when time permitted. Now, I felt I could barely contemplate walking around the garden because I was so physically weak. It did not help to know that, whenever I *was* able to return to gardening, I would have to be so much more careful. I felt too young to be having such restrictions placed on my life and this was reinforced for me when, during my early convalescence, a friend took me for a gentle walk to pick some blackberries. I had no gloves and had to be *so* careful to protect my left arm from scratches that hitherto I would not even have thought about.

As far as the garden was concerned, I was blessed by my own, personal 'Ground Farce' as my husband dubbed them! Two close friends came regularly to work in our back garden, to ensure that, when weather permitted, it would be a good place to sit. Sometimes they were hard at work before I was even up. Often, I would sit outside and talk to them as they worked, occasionally fetching and carrying a little. It was so generous of them to give their time like that to do what I could not. I could never repay that kindness but I hope that they know and understand the pleasure it gave me to look at their handiwork. They gave me practical help and enduring enjoyment – the perfect gift in the circumstances.

Healing seemed a fairly slow process. I had had two general anaesthetics in fairly quick succession and I suppose that didn't help. Friends, particularly those from the music ministry and from work, were very conscientious about visiting me to lend support and to help the time to pass. I had to heal for two weeks before I would visit the clinic to receive the histology report, meet the oncologist and plan to begin my chemotherapy. There would then be a further two weeks before the chemotherapy could actually begin.

At around this time, I had to visit the breast clinic to have my staples removed. This was when I actually learned that there were forty-two in all; I took them home and counted them. The nurse who removed them was skilled and gentle and she remarked, 'That's neat!' referring to my scar, as she worked. I was not able to admire the new state of my chest as she had done. I was still feeling pretty raw about my 'new' body. I told her, 'I'm glad you think so!' Martin, my husband, who was sitting watching, said, 'Well you've only seen *your* scar, but the nurse has seen hundreds.' At this the nurse, whose name was Kerry, paused in her work to say, 'Yes, including my own.' Now I was hungry for details.

This inspiring lady told me that breast cancer had hit her after she had recovered from another cancer in her digestive tract. She had been through mastectomy and chemotherapy. She spoke of her depression when she had to attend what had once been her place of work as a patient and how she had then been inclined to tears at the thought that she would never return there in her professional capacity. Now here she was, fully restored to health and assuring me that there really was light at the end of this tunnel. What comfort I drew from her words and her quiet courage in sharing with me her most vulnerable experiences! She helped me so much that day, and whenever I have seen her since, I have found her to be a tonic. Her experiences have made of her a truly gifted nurse and I feel sure that her presence at that time was God's gift of reassurance to me.

Another issue was raised at about this time which was a difficult one to consider, and it was partly due to me that it came up at all. I had perforce had much time to think about the circumstances of my diagnosis and I was anxious. After all, the G.P. hadn't spotted the cancer in my left breast, so how did we know that the right breast was O.K.? The surgeon assured me that they had examined it very thoroughly and that was comforting to know. Now I wanted to know something else. If I decided to have my left breast reconstructed, I knew the right breast would have to be reduced – but how would that affect the detection of any future cancer in that breast?

The answer, when it came, was *not* comforting. Basically, because of the presence of scar tissue, detection would be much more difficult. So here was the deal: as things stood, I had this very large right breast, which had already undergone minor surgeries for benign lumps, in which the tissues were fibrous and dense, and from experience I knew that cancer would be difficult to detect, should it develop there. If I had the breast reduced, cancer would be even more difficult to detect. And there was a feeling that, even if I didn't want reconstruction, I may have to go for a reduction just in order to achieve a really satisfactory and manageable result with a prosthesis… The surgeon, perhaps sensing and echoing my fears, jumped straight in with his suggestion; once I had been through chemo and any other necessary treatment, if I wished to consider the prophylactic removal of the right breast, he would be happy to arrange it. Following that, he would build two small 'blind' breasts for me (without nipples), possibly about A cup size, using my own skin and muscle tissue. Much later, I found out that, partly because of the size of the breasts I had lost, this particular reconstruction solution was unlikely ever to be successful...

Obviously, to some extent, the surgeon shared my worry about detecting any future cancer. He even told me to remember that there would be no guarantees after the other breast was removed, as statistics have shown that surgeons leave behind between five and fifteen percent of breast tissue, as he had once told me. Clearly, I needed to think carefully about my options.

It didn't take long. My husband and I talked it over in the car on the way home. By the time we arrived, we had *both* decided that there was really only one option; if the surgeon was still happy to do it when the time came, I would have the other breast removed and both breasts rebuilt, using my own body tissues. There were no considerations this time over anything as seemingly unimportant as nipple sensitivity...

The histology report when it came was, in a way, a non-event because, thankfully, it showed up no new problems; it simply confirmed what was already known about my situation. The surgical consultant was beaming as he told me that there were no further complications and I would not need radiotherapy. 'Thank God!' I thought, and I meant it. It was not so much the radiotherapy that I dreaded, but the long, daily drive to a distant hospital where it would be administered. My heart singing with the joy of having been relieved of this threat, I set off to see the oncologist...

A number of oncologists work together in our hospital, and I met a young, gentle lady doctor with a very sweet bedside manner, who carefully explained to me that they were intending to attack my cancer in three specific ways. They would use hormone therapy by continuing the Tamoxifen as a daily dose. As I have said before, my tumour had been mildly oestrogen dependent and heavily progestogen dependent, so, she explained, taking Tamoxifen to block oestrogen would help, because we have a bio-feedback system in our bodies, with the rise and fall of levels of hormones depending on each other. Therefore, blocking oestrogen would do some good in itself but it would also result in a drop in progestogen. It looked as if I would be taking the pills for a very long time...

Next, the doctor talked about the chemotherapy. As the patient, you keep waiting for a break – the bit of good news that you weren't expecting. At the time of the first histology report, I had wanted to hear that the tumour hadn't invaded my lymph nodes – but it had. I had wanted to hear that my tumour was not heavily invasive – but it was. Now I wanted to hear that I did not have to have the aggressive chemotherapy and that I would not lose my hair. No such luck. The doctor explained that I would need what she called FEC chemotherapy, a combination of three drugs, each having a catalogue of side effects that would make your toes curl to read it! Oh well, I thought, at least it will be over more quickly, because I thought (though as I have said before, I may well have been mistaken) the breast care nurse had told me that patients on the more aggressive chemotherapy usually only had to endure four cycles, whereas those on the gentler one had to have six. Not so. The doctor was now explaining to me that research showed that there was a much better outcome for patients like myself if they had *six* cycles of FEC chemo. Oh dear!

There was worse to come, and I knew that break definitely wasn't coming my way at this point, when she explained that the third part of my treatment plan was to be radiotherapy. *WHAT? Hadn't the other doctor just told me I wouldn't need it? Hadn't my heart been singing with gratitude at that news?*

Gently, seeing my shock and distress, the doctor explained that she, the cancer specialist, was in a better position than my surgeon to determine whether I needed radiotherapy or not, and that studies had shown that people in my position did better when they had radiotherapy treatment – and not just treatment to the chest wall; they were planning to irradiate my neck as well, to mop up any stray cancer cells that might be lingering there in lymph nodes.

So, I *was* to have radiotherapy, and not just to one site but to two. At the time, this was almost too much to bear. I had been so relieved to be told that I didn't need it. The tears came. The doctor was very understanding and very patient. She seemed to wonder if I was rejecting the treatment plan she was offering. I quickly assured her that whatever she felt was necessary, I was prepared to do. Perhaps, at this point, I suffered because I was not able to 'let go and let God'. I have always been a person who likes to be in control; possibly this is due to some deep-seated insecurities. Looking back at this time, I know that the treatment plan was right. I simply had some difficulty in adjusting my frame of mind to this at the time: 'Be patient; God hasn't finished with me yet!' as I've sometimes seen written on T-shirts!

I was given a careful physical examination. Particular attention was paid to the remaining breast and to my upper tummy. I felt I had guessed what the oncologist's agenda was and I begged her please not to find any tumours on my liver. She grinned and said it felt fine. The consultation did not end until the doctor felt that I fully understood what I needed to know about the chemotherapy (which was to be the next phase of my treatment), and was calm. Then I was taken down the corridor to the chemo clinic where an appointment for the following week was booked for me. At that appointment my height would be measured and I would be weighed in order to determine the dosage I should be given when my drugs would be administered the following week.

I would need to buy a wig. I was definitely going to lose my hair and I'm not a person who can wear hats. My hair was in very good condition because I had resisted the temptation to use chemical treatments and I took great care of it. It was long (halfway down my back), soft and gleaming. I rang my hairdresser and made an appointment to have it cut. I had not worn my hair short for about eighteen years. My husband had always said how much he liked it long, and in any case I suppose I felt that long hair was part of the uniform for a female folk/rhythm guitarist. Once again, the image that I liked to show to the world was about to take a severe knock – just one more aspect of the stripping exercise I had felt I was undergoing before surgery. Without this experience, perhaps I would have hidden behind my image for the rest of my days. As it was, not only was I forced to confront my real self, but others joined me in my vulnerability. This proved to be an honest and enriching experience.

My hairdresser was great. Not only did she cut my hair very short, but she chose a free and easy style that I actually quite liked. She also gave me very good advice on the best place to purchase a wig (apparently the price is much the same whether you buy from the NHS or privately) and directions on how to get there. Later the same day I saw my friends at our weekly prayer meeting and was amazed at how much people obviously and genuinely liked my new image.

The next day Martin and I went wig shopping. We found the recommended store without difficulty and were directed to the department. It was tucked away at the side of the store and had a small range of hairpieces of various kinds on display around the entrance to a little fitting booth designed to give privacy. This was misleading, as I thought there could hardly be much of a range of choice in such a small space with an apparently limited display. I was in for a surprise.

The lady in attendance there was a real sweetheart. She ascertained that I would like to look as much myself as possible and set about gathering items for me to try on. Of course hygiene is important in such circumstances so I was given a kind of skull cap to wear over my now short hair in order to try on the wigs. My hair, however, was very clean and shiny and the skull cap just wouldn't stay in place but began to creep towards the crown of my head ready to 'ping' off at the first opportunity! This was a problem, because I was constantly aware of these strange creeping sensations and did not know that it was the skull cap, made of the same sort of fabric as tights, and not the wig that was responsible. All I knew was that something wasn't sitting tight and I felt neither comfortable nor confident. Eventually the assistant realised that the wretched thing just wasn't going to stay put, and on the basis that I had washed my hair that morning and that it hadn't yet started to fall out because I hadn't yet had my first chemo treatment, we abandoned any attempt to cover my hair first and just put the wigs straight onto my head.

I tried on at least about seven or eight wigs, all of which roughly approximated to my new, short hairstyle. I was encouraged, whilst wearing each one in turn, to walk to the window and view myself in a mirror by daylight. That way I would have a really clear idea about colour. There were two wigs that both Martin and I liked. One was a really close match for my own hair, aside from having a permanent parting. The other was very similar, but had blonde highlights, something I had not risked since my teens! Martin really liked it. I think it had something to do with the fact that he was very keen on Tina Turner at the time and there was something about this highlighted wig which slightly reflected her leonine mane – despite it being much tamer! Anyhow, we bought the plain one…and a week later, I went back and bought the highlights as well! Well, if you're going to have to endure being bald, you might as well have what fun you can – and in any case, and on a more serious note, acrylic wigs are really easily damaged by heat, say from opening the oven door, and my husband was concerned that if I only had one wig and I damaged it I might be somewhat compromised. I really appreciated his generosity with the family funds. Incidentally, if you're thinking about real hair, forget it, unless you've upwards of £500 to spare and you want to spend a lot of time and money taking care of your wig. I have to say that both of my acrylic wigs look very good – but, oh boy, did I miss the feel and behaviour of my own real hair once I had none!

I wore the new wig briefly – the one I purchased first – on a couple of occasions before I lost my hair, to show it to my close friends, who were impressed because it looked so natural. On one of these occasions, my son came in and immediately my friend signalled that I should say nothing. My son didn't notice that I was wearing the wig, even though he looked closely at me several times. As the adults present began to get the giggles, he stroppily asked what was so funny. (Not at all unreasonable, because we had made him feel uncomfortable; he knew we were keeping something from him.) We told him, and digesting the news with good grace, he responded that I was 'going to look O.K.' Coming from him, and thus passing the teenage credibility test, this did me the world of good, but there is definitely no substitute for one's own hair, however good the wig, and I was to miss mine terribly in due course.

One day, during the run up to the chemotherapy, we received a phone call from our daughter, along the lines of, 'I'm on my way home. Please can Dad pick me up from the station? And, by the way, I've got a surprise for you.' Martin ruefully said to me, 'I hope this surprise is one I can stomach!' Anyone who has ever raised teenagers will know exactly what he meant. Anyhow, he left for the station and shortly returned with our daughter in tow. She had had her head completely shaved. Gone were the curls and the ponytail. Now she sported a number one clipper cut which accentuated the neat and attractive lines of her skull. 'I did it first so that you wouldn't have to be afraid,' she said. 'It's really not so scary.' And then she threw herself into my arms and we cried together. All her life my daughter has favoured long hair. She's the hair ornament queen, is my Lizzy. She spends a fortune on her locks – treatments, perms, weaves, extensions – and now here she was, completely shorn. What could I say in response to such a gesture? I just hugged her very tight. It was an occasion that my heart will always treasure, reflecting on the generosity of hers.

And so the chemotherapy began. Both Martin and Lizzy came with me for my first treatment, to offer moral support. Chemotherapy at our local hospital takes place in a room the size of a good domestic lounge. In that room are about four or so easy chairs, each with a pillow on one arm. The decor is attractive and lounge-like; the chair covers are chintzy. The patient sits in one of the armchairs and has the undivided attention of a nurse on a one-to-one basis during the treatment. I sat in my allotted armchair and Lizzy and Martin, who were allowed in to keep me company, sat on high-backed dining chairs positioned against a wall. The nurse introduced herself, encouraging me to address her by her first name, and then began to explain in careful detail what was to happen. I was to be hooked up to a drip containing saline. Once that was successfully up and running, the various drugs would be administered through a valve in the drip line, one syringe at a time. My arm would rest on the pillow.

First I was given a syringe of a clear fluid, which I was told was an anti-sickness drug. The main side effect of chemotherapy is nausea, though there are many others worthy of note! This first syringe was of the size you might usually associate with 'jabs' – an average-looking piece of medical kit. The second was markedly smaller and I was told that it contained a little dose of a steroid. The job of this steroid was to potentiate, to make stronger or more effective, the anti-sickness drug I had just received. Remember, these things were not going in through needles, just straight into the drip to which I was already attached. So far, so good.

Now came the big guns; the three drugs that were prescribed for my particular kind of chemotherapy. The first was a drug called Fluorouracil which was a clear fluid in a huge (honestly!) plastic syringe. This was fed slowly into the drip and was closely followed by a similar sized dose of Epirubicin, which is a strange, red fluid, then Cyclophosphamide, another clear fluid. I do not jest when I say that the syringes holding these fluids are huge, and I would advise anyone who is about to undergo chemotherapy to visit the toilet beforehand unless they are very sure of a generous bladder capacity. Fluid in, in my experience, equals fluid out!

As well as having a wide range of well documented side effects, these drugs have certain immediate effects on the body, noticeable even as they are gently pushed into the feed line. One gives a very strange and prickly sensation in the nose and sinuses. Another gives a strange and prickly sensation 'down under'. One makes you feel slightly drunk – as if, perhaps you've had a glass or two of wine on an empty stomach – and as soon as you go to the loo after Epirubicin, you'll discover that your urine has become an alarming red-orange shade! All of these things I was warned about by the nurse, as well as other possible side effects I may experience. The chemo process did not hurt, nor did I feel particularly ill – rather, I would say, it made me feel somehow *alien* and not quite myself, odd as that sounds. This was a little alarming, but I must say that the nurses in attendance were extremely attentive, calm and reassuring, which helped a great deal.

Chemotherapy works by interfering with the way that cancer cells reproduce – interfering with cell division. Cells that are affected become damaged and eventually die. Different drugs interfere with this process in different ways and that is why it is necessary to take more than one such drug. Unfortunately, it is not only cancerous cells that the drugs affect. Healthy cells needed by the body that happen to be dividing at that time are also hit, and the consequences can be severe.

The administration of the chemo takes between half an hour and forty-five minutes, after which the drip is removed and the patient allowed to leave. During the treatment everything possible is done to make the patient comfortable and to facilitate the process. For example, I have very difficult veins, so my arm was soaked in warm water before the drip was connected; also, some patients experience a bad taste in their mouth as the drugs are administered and they are offered a drink or a boiled sweet to suck. The atmosphere is always calm and caring.

After the chemotherapy treatment I was to see the doctor, the lady oncologist, again. We moved, therefore, to join her queue on a different area of corridor and sat among many whom I had met in hospital when I had my surgery, to await our turn. I had a minor but pressing matter to discuss with her. Two months before I knew I had breast cancer, I had seen another consultant at the hospital to investigate pelvic pain. I had had a cystoscopy to look inside the bladder, just in case I might be developing disease there, and that had not revealed any problem. The consultant had told me that he wanted me to have a non-urgent laparoscopy to look inside my tummy using a tiny camera to view my reproductive organs because my uterus was bulky. Now a bulky uterus is not unusual in a woman of forty-eight who is beginning the menopause but one of the known side effects of Tamoxifen, the hormone-blocking drug that I was now taking every day, is that it can cause the lining of the womb, the endometrium, to thicken, causing a bulky uterus, and it has also been implicated in uterine cancer; yes, the drug you take to stave off your breast cancer can give you cancer of the womb! Because I knew that there was a possibility that all was not right 'down there' even before all this began, I now felt particularly at risk.

I had talked to the breast care nurse about this surgery for which I was on a waiting list, and she had suggested that I write to the gynaecological consultant who had ordered it. In my letter, she said, I should explain my present circumstances. Perhaps a minor operation such as this could take place during my chemotherapy if it was carefully timed. Accordingly, I had written the letter and now I needed to inform the lady oncologist, who agreed that the surgery would be possible, with careful timing and appropriate precautions. I must, she said, inform the oncology team as soon as I received a proposed date for the procedure. We thanked her and left.

The days after that first chemo session were a voyage of discovery. The drug I had been given against sickness and the pills I had been given to take at home worked very well. They did not take away all nausea, but I was never sick. However, they have a notorious side effect – constipation – and having suffered (*really* suffered) from that after my last bout of surgery because of the pain-killers I'd been on, I definitely didn't want to go *there* again! I ate enormous amounts of vegetable stew, regardless of my appetite, which was limited. I was also taking golden linseeds on a daily basis, as advised by the book I have mentioned before. I found the advice I gleaned from that book invaluable, particularly with regard to nutrition whilst on chemotherapy. Thanks to Professor Jane Plant, I was juicing carrots, apples and broccoli daily. (She added fennel to her apple juice, but I added broccoli to mine because she explains that it contains powerful anti-cancer agents that are destroyed by cooking and I found it easier to drink the juice than to eat broccoli every day!) As well as this, I aimed to eat my meals, regardless of appetite, ensuring that I had a wide range of fruit and vegetables daily and I avoided all dairy produce, substituting soya products in their place as she advises. Broccoli juice is very strong and frankly horrible and only bearable when diluted by adding it to the apple juice. It is too strong to drink without dilution, at least with water, in any case, but I was drinking my juices, eating my vegetables, taking vitamins A, C and E and selenium, swallowing brewers' yeast and red clover – trying hard to do my bit. I believe that God leads us to helpful information; we then need to make use of it, proceeding prayerfully. In the event, in one way at least, I overdid it, because I had to get up three times in that first night after the chemo to go to the loo! So much for working to avoid constipation!

I have mentioned before that the chemo made me feel 'alien' and I still think that that is the best description. I did not feel ill in those early stages, I felt strange and somehow other-worldly. This phase lasted for three days. During this time, my sleep pattern was particularly disturbed – a side effect of the steroids taken to boost the anti-sickness drug. Friends found it amazing that, though I could and often did, sleep during the day, I could be wide awake and hyper at one a.m.! One friend, who was also on chemotherapy, described this condition perfectly: 'Your head is saying, 'Let's go to sleep,' but your legs are saying, 'No, let's go for a good run around the block'.' I knew just what she meant. There is a strange combination of mental weariness and physical hyperactivity involved. The steroids also impaired my ability both to think clearly and to articulate my thoughts; sometimes I felt I was almost tripping over my own mouth! (This is a condition I've also known when well; the Lord is working on my 'foot in mouth disease', but I assure you this time it was different!)

As time progressed, in later chemotherapy cycles, this problem with talking sense became a particular irritation to me, because I had always been a competent and relatively confident speaker. Now the parts inside of me that used to facilitate that skill couldn't always get it together and I found that hard to cope with. However, once these particular pills were out of my system on the first occasion, things thankfully gradually returned to normal in these respects. In later cycles I was to discover that many such side effects would become more persistent. On the fourth day of this first cycle I just felt a bit wobbly, but on the fifth things went rather downhill. I almost fainted in the bathroom and had to be assisted into bed. I felt suddenly so very weak, yet I had only been bathing.

During chemotherapy, the levels of certain types of blood cells will take a nose-dive, usually between the seventh day and the tenth, I was told, and at that point, you will feel weak and need to rest as the body dictates – and that was pretty much the way that it was that first time through. The eleventh day (and the night just before it) was awful. Overnight I seemed incapable of regulating my body temperature. I shivered and could not sleep. During the day, I felt that I had suddenly become very old and very slow. I felt dreadful and I was told that I looked it! I was to discover that, throughout the chemo treatment, I would often have trouble in regulating my body temperature. One moment I would be freezing, my fingers white with Reynaud's syndrome (from which I have always suffered) and bloodless, the next my shivers would be replaced by unbearable hot flushes, thanks either to the menopause or Tamoxifen, or both. However, by the next day in cycle one, that phase had passed, and though I felt a little fragile, I was much better – just as well, really, as I was due to play guitar in church.

Essentially, our music ministry has a core of three people, two who play guitar and sing and one who sings and plays percussion. Friends who are perhaps parts of other music ministries often join us; we are very close to some of them and many have been wonderful support to me during my illness. On Sundays, the three of us were, at this time, usually joined by a schoolgirl who played the flute, so the usual number playing at church was four. On this particular Sunday, John, the lead guitarist, rang in the morning to tell me that he was terribly sorry, but he wouldn't be able to play at church that afternoon. His disabled sister was to make a rare visit to his home and he needed to be there for her. Clearly, this was the priority. Those who have daily charge of his sister (who lives in a care home) had spoken to me in the past of the way her face lights up just because this brother of hers enters the room. How could he not be there when she made a rare visit to his home? I told him that he was absolutely right to stay at home, and not to worry, but I knew that he felt torn. He would dearly have liked to be able to be in two places at once! In myself, I was concerned. I felt well but fragile, having been so very unwell the day before. But the other two would be there, and I had been the only guitarist on other occasions when circumstances demanded it; it was something that, under normal circumstances, I was quite used to. I spoke to my husband, who agreed to take me early to church so that I wouldn't have to rush. We decided to take two guitars because I felt it would be just like me to break a string when there was no one there for back-up!

Now, I have mentioned before in this account how I had become so very aware that God was providing for me and for others, but on this day in particular, I had an astounding proof of divine providence in the truest sense: God literally providing for me. During the previous year, when we had played fortnightly for the healing prayer group in London, we had often been joined by a young couple, themselves a music ministry, who enjoyed singing and playing with us. The husband is an accomplished guitarist and he and his wife both sing. Because the young man preferred my second guitar to his own, he had regularly played it and was very comfortable with it. This couple lived in London, whereas we live further to the north, some miles from the capital, in Essex.

About six months before this particular Sunday, they had left their London home to begin a new life as the resident music ministry in a Christian community in Liverpool. We had not seen them since. Now, just as mass was starting, they walked into our Essex church. I do not think they had ever been there before; indeed, I could not think what they were doing there now, though I was extremely grateful for their presence! They had a female friend with them. I asked the young man if he would like to play guitar. He said yes, as I knew he would, and picked up my faithful Fender, with which he was so familiar. His wife and their friend sat in a nearby pew and sang. The music fell easily into place because we were so used to playing together, and I was absolved from the responsibility of being a solo guitarist. Though I sat for much of the proceedings, I was not unwell. After the mass, we asked this couple how they came to be there.

It transpired that they had returned to London the previous day to see to the selling of their flat in a north London district. They were now on their return journey to Liverpool, but had looked for a mass to attend, between somewhere and South Woodford (I have forgotten what the other district they named was) and had picked this one from a directory. Of all the churches in London and Essex, they had walked into ours; and of all the possible mass times available, they had chosen the one we would be attending, at the somewhat unusual time of four-thirty in the afternoon! Had they known we would be there? No. The wife had apparently said to her husband as they drew up outside the church that she had an idea that this might be the one where we played on Sundays, but he had thought she was mistaken. In any case, they would not have known the time that we would be due to be there; a different choir is there in the mornings. They had no knowledge either of my illness, shocked to discover the reason I had chosen to sit and so pleased that they had been brought to help. They were as surprised and delighted by this 'God-incidence' as we were, and there was much hugging and sharing of news.

After the mass when we returned home, I rang John. I was so full of gratitude to God, so amazed at this provision for us. It had been totally right for him to be at home, for and with his family, during that afternoon, and God had covered for that in the most extraordinary way, using our friends from 'up north'. He was just as amazed and delighted as I had been. Much of our conversation was conducted in raised voices and exclamations figured greatly in the vocabulary between us. Perhaps we should not be surprised that God cares for our needs so well – but I was totally elated for at least two days afterwards, every time I recalled this particular gift. The circumstances were so remarkable that I do not think it possible to explain away the apparent coincidence; God was at work here, and that is that!

Since the first dose of chemotherapy had been administered, I had been working very hard, as I said before, at my personal nutrition, taking supplements and drinking juices. I felt well in myself and a decision was made that, since the school where I was employed was open to staff only during this particular week (no pupils), it would be safe, and probably very good for me, to attend the meetings and planning sessions that were taking place. Despite my nutritional efforts, however, my hair began to fall out as they had said it would. At first it was nothing too traumatic; I would put up my hand to my head and bring down five or so hairs – but each day the number increased until, on the morning I was due to return to school, there was a major, dramatic event; I took a shower! In itself, totally unremarkable, I know, but then it is not usual to step out from under the shower and find that you have left a complete carpet of human hair in the bathtub. Not all of my hair had fallen out, but clearly the process was well underway, and I felt it would have been just plain anti-social to have gone anywhere until I could be sure I wouldn't leave a trail of hair behind me.

I shrieked for Martin. The poor man came at a run, took in the bathtub and its contents, and became, as so often before, a pillar of strength. We had decided that, when this moment came, he would shave my head and I would wear the wig from that moment on. We rang the school to tell them of my unavoidable delay. Martin fetched the clippers, led me downstairs, spread newspapers on the living room floor, and gently sat me down. I sat there on the newsprint carpet, watching what was left of my hair cascading to the floor around me. It was somehow surreal. He worked steadily and methodically, declaring that he didn't want anything patchy; he wanted to get it right.

When he had finished, he took me back to the bathroom to shave my neck, since my hairline tends to be rather low – something that had never bothered me when I wore my hair long. I confronted my new self in the mirror. There was no denying his professionalism; he had done a good job indeed, but I can't say I liked what I saw. My daughter, as I have said, had shaved her head. Her skull underneath was a wonderful shape that flattered her face. Mine was more of an egg, or even a potato, I felt, and did nothing for my face, blessed as I was with a square jaw and a double chin, but there was nothing to be done but get on with life, so I fetched the wig and put it on.

For the first hour or thereabouts, I felt as if I was wearing a hat. I had a tendency to look out from under the wig and my husband had to remind me to hold my head up. I've never, as I said, been a hat person. On the whole, they don't suit me. I didn't even wear a veil when we married; just flowers on a band in my long hair. Now I was condemned to wear what was effectively a hat of hair for at least six months – or be bald.

I learnt to live with it pretty quickly and was at school before mid-day. I cannot speak highly enough of the head teacher or my colleagues. All were universally supportive and very complimentary about the hair – even some who had not been told about my situation and who just assumed I'd had a makeover! They really hadn't known that the hair was not my own. Thus my confidence in at least this aspect of my appearance grew…but I saw myself regularly in the bedroom mirror in the days that followed, and there is no denying that it was hard. 'God looked at what He had made and saw that it was good'. I looked at what the cancer had done to me… I was bald. I had a long scar where my left breast had been and the area of skin beneath it was like crepe. My right breast, hanging large and alone, looked to me somehow ludicrous. I was some strange, new thing to look at, yet people constantly assured me that I was still myself…Well, maybe so, but this self took some coming to terms with. Sometimes, when I fell asleep, I had dreams about having hair… And I truly did – indeed, I *do* – believe that if He wished to do it because it was right for me, God could make me a new breast – just like that – so once, after praying, I looked for it… I was always open to the possibility that it may happen, though I never doubted that if it did not, then there was a very good reason; maybe I was learning something I needed to take on board – patience, for example! More likely there were things that I needed to experience in order to gain new insights or skills. I had to know that God was at work in His wisdom, which is far beyond mine!

One real downside of not being a 'hat person'? Well, during chemotherapy treatment, I was to discover that a bald head can be very cold in bed at night! As a result of feeling the chill

I had to resort to wearing a blue woolly hat that my son had previously owned and worn at age three! (It was very easily stretched!) This I alternated with a white woolly baby hat that some friends kindly picked up for me, having checked that it, too, 'had plenty of stretch'. In one or other of these, then, I nightly retired, feeling, with hat and missing a breast, about as sexy as a doormat. It had its funny side…

There came a night when, for some reason I have forgotten, both of these hats were in the wash together and I was desperate for warm headgear. Now both of our children are of dual heritage and both have, at times, experimented with braids and locks. One Christmas when they were still quite small, I had made for each of them an orange and yellow woolly hat with long black braids and fringes attached, trimmed at the ends with the same orange and yellow yarn. They had worn these for some time, with pride and delight, and in fact the hats had often fooled members of the general public who had clearly believed they were viewing the children's hair, until perhaps the hat was whisked off due to the child being uncomfortably hot in a crowded bus or tube, causing hilarity all around. Now here I was, with a cold head and no hat, and only these two available. I put one on, and went to bed. I do not, it must be admitted, have the face for that hat. The children used to look great in them. They have been known to don them recently, just to recall the fun. In my state of post chemo pastiness the black braids were not exactly flattering. My husband came up to tuck me in and split his sides. Ah well…

My daughter's closest companion (now her partner) had also been kind enough to give me a large number of headscarves. These I found very useful from time to time; especially one which was made of soft cotton. I wore them around the house, but had to stop wearing them to bed quite early in my 'bald phase' as my head became very sensitive to pressure, and scarves can tend to fall into ridges. Nevertheless, I made grateful use of them for a long while.

So once the 'Great Head Shaving Event' was over, I went in to work that day as I had planned to do. I had three great days at school, during which I really felt able to contribute to the meetings and I also benefited from the information I absorbed from the carefully presented update sessions for all staff. It was a strange thing to be in some ways fully involved with what had previously been my working world and yet in others to feel slightly removed, unable to forget what was going on elsewhere in my life, and unsure as to what the outcome might be. Also, it was impossible to forget that I was only there because the children were not. I am a teacher, after all, and my working place is in front of a class, yet this was not going to be possible for a very long time. I couldn't even cope with three full days in school at meetings; on two of those days I had to quit at midday or shortly after. I worried about the impression this would give. Would people think me a freeloader, along for the bits of the ride that I fancied? Yet, when I came home because of tiredness, I could go straight to bed at two in the afternoon and fall instantly to sleep.

Straight after those three days I had to have a blood test as a routine precaution before my second chemotherapy session, due later that week. It was not a pleasant procedure – they never are for me; as I have told you, I have very difficult veins and now I only had one available arm. Eventually, the man who first tried to get my blood passed me over to an older man who managed to draw blood from the back of my hand, using a thing designed for children, and therefore having smaller dimensions, a 'paediatric butterfly'. Of one thing, however, I was supremely confident. My blood would be great! The nurses at the clinic would be asking how I managed to have such super levels of all the requisite cells while on chemotherapy. I would tell everyone all about my nutrition regime and the juicing I was doing, and they'd all be impressed. They might even want to start giving other patients similar dietary recommendations, I thought, because I'd worked so hard at eating all the right things and everyone said I looked so well. I was so proud of my efforts…

…And pride comes before a fall, as everyone knows.

I was out shopping for organic food when the phone-call came. There was a fuel crisis on, so Martin and I had walked to the supermarket to save petrol and share the carrying of the load. I had done three days in school and I was feeling both good and confident; after all, I was working a little and walking fair distances, so what could be wrong? As we walked through the side door, our son broke the news. 'Mum, the hospital phoned and said not to go for your chemo tomorrow. They said your blood's not right or something.'

I reacted very badly. This simply couldn't be. First I raved. Then I got on the phone to the hospital. The chemo nurses were polite but firm. I could not have my chemotherapy because I was neutropenic; the level of neutrophil blood cells in my body had fallen dangerously low, meaning that I was at great risk of succumbing to infection if I was exposed, because these cells are an important part of the body's defence system. If chemotherapy was administered in such circumstances, they told me, I would almost certainly end up in hospital being reverse barrier nursed. I knew what that meant. I had seen people on the breast ward who were, because they had caught an infection that they couldn't fight without help, confined to a single room for their own protection, with limited visitors who had to wear aprons or gowns in order to enter the room. The object of the exercise is to fight the infection aggressively and protect the patient from the danger of exposure to any other nasty organisms.

I simply didn't believe this news. I felt good, and I had just completed time at work. It could not be that, after all our efforts to get the right food into me and all that juicing and fish (the last at the specific request of the lady oncologist that I must have some omega 3 fish oils in my diet), I was less than healthy! I queried the blood results again and was told that it was not as if I was borderline; I was 'way down'. What could I do, I asked? What should I have done that I hadn't? I had been so pleased with myself, so sure that I was a star performer, and now this.

Apparently there was nothing I could have done. Chemotherapy wipes out these little white cells along with any cancer cells. Your body then makes new ones, but each person's body does this at its own rate. The cells are very important because they are needed to help the body fight bacterial infection; they have little effect on viral things, such as colds. No amount of careful diet or effort at good living was likely to affect my body's ability to renew these little warriors; it was doing the best it could and we would just have to wait. I would have another blood test the next week, and if that showed improvement, I would have my chemo then.

Now I was really fed up. We had worked so hard to keep me well, the sole aim being to have all the treatments on time and get to the end of the chemo as early as possible. I had worked out the minimum time it need take and I was aiming for, *focussed on*, that. I had not even contemplated the possibility of setbacks, because my routine was going to show the world how these things should be successfully tackled; I was going to lead the way for others! And now, at only the second cycle of my chemo,

I was in a backwater with nothing to do but wait. Worse, I was warned that I was severely at risk of infection – had been for days, *including those three days in school* – and I must be careful and must monitor my temperature daily. 'Wonderwoman' became the fragile flower that needed protecting. How could this be? I railed at the chemotherapy nurse. What was the point, I asked her, in all my efforts – all that juicing, all those swallowed supplements – if it couldn't stop this from happening? I would just stop all that now, because it was darned hard work and there was clearly no point! Patiently she told me that I knew that wasn't true: I must keep up my efforts, must do what I could to fight the disease.

I rang the school and told them that I wouldn't be in for a while. I rang my dad. Disappointed as I was, he was as ever wise, supportive and philosophical. Despite (or maybe because of) his previous encounters with the disease, he had been from the point of my diagnosis an unfailing source of strength. He had helped to keep me going with wise words and enormous faith and fortitude – not to mention his skilfully crafted poems, full of his trust in God and his love for me and tailor made to my circumstances, which had arrived in a steady trickle through the post at the times when they were most needed. In the end, we acknowledged, I simply had to accept this. God knows best, even when Helen is only able to admit this through gritted teeth!

From the first, my husband and my father had been steadfast in their loving support. My husband's parents had been unstinting in their efforts to reassure me of their great love, their devastation at the news of my illness and their desire to 'be there' in any way possible, as had his siblings. Also my brother, a clinical doctor of pharmacy living at that time in New Zealand with his lovely wife, had gone out of his way to telephone, to reassure (and his reassurances meant a great deal because I knew that he 'knew his stuff') and to urge me ever forward toward recovery. He was constant in his encouragement, telling me truthfully that around half the patients in my position not only get well, but they never have another brush with the disease; even those whose disease recurs usually have many years first when things are successfully under control. He was helpful in restoring hope. My sisters, two in Birmingham and one in New Zealand, kept in constant, faithful touch and were also always helpful and reassuring, as were Martin's siblings and many members of our wider families.

Helpful also at this time was the male friend with whom I play guitar. Hearing about my deferred chemo and my downheartedness, he would not countenance any threats to quit my healthy eating regime. He simply confronted me; I *knew* I had to make those efforts. I *knew* any talk of stopping was wild and crazy. I just had to continue to do what I could to help myself, and this situation, disappointing as it was, hadn't really changed a thing. I must get on with it! 'Cut the crap,' in other words! As a talented businessman, skilled in sales, he wasn't going to allow my blatant emotionalism to sabotage a potential good deal! He and his sound and practical wife pinned me in love and solid good sense.

It was, however, my other close friend (the one who herself worked in the hospital and who had sung with me for nine years) who hit the nail uncomfortably on the head. She pointed out that, from the start, there had been a fundamental error in my approach to this whole scenario. God had given me various means to help myself in fighting this disease, but I had been inclined to believe that these things somehow meant that I was in control. Maybe I needed this setback to remind me that Almighty God (and not Helen with her juicing machine!)

was in the driving seat. (Just as well, really, as I was already on my third juicing machine – this one semi-industrial – after 'thraping' two others within weeks in my efforts to consume juices at a rate they couldn't match.) And so, at last, I had to accept (or begin to accept, for the journey to acceptance is a long process) that I would have to take things at the pace that God, and not I, dictated.

The next day I had an appointment for a fitting with a proper prosthesis. At least problems with the quality of my blood wouldn't get in the way of that! I was looking forward to being given my long term false breast. When I left hospital I had been given two 'comfy' prostheses, one to wash and one to wear. These had been simply those soft white cotton envelopes, oval shaped, stuffed with the kind of material used in duvets or children's toys. I had not found them entirely satisfactory and I had sent by mail order for a foam breast form which I had found a little better. At the same time as ordering the foam breast form I had ordered a 'sleep bra'. The reason for this was my lack of confidence. I was very worried that either we may have visitors staying at our house, or we would, for example, visit family, and they would be confronted with the one-breasted woman in her nightclothes! At the time, the thought of this really troubled me, and the catalogues promised that this garment was devised to prevent just such eventualities, having a pocket to hold the breast form in place, but being soft enough to sleep in. Great, I thought, I'd order one and my confidence would be restored.

Women who have mastectomies come in all sizes, right? So why don't sleep bras? Is it that women with small ribcages and big boobs are somehow not in *need* of the same confidence boosts as anyone else? The wretched garment was not available in **my** size. Why not? I suppose it just isn't cost effective to mass produce something that wouldn't fit the majority of women. Sighing, I asked the girl on the phone to send me a sleep bra that would accommodate the breast form she thought I would need and *I* would make it fit my ribcage. I sew quite well and I did manage to make the thing fit me after a fashion, but I never wore that sleep bra. However, I used the foam prosthesis, even though it was on the small side, from the day of its arrival until the day of my fitting at clinic.

As I had said, the quality of my blood couldn't prevent my attending the fitting clinic – but the fuel crisis prevented the *fitting specialist* from attending! She was just as vital to that appointment as any nurse – more, really, because in this field she *is* the specialist, but she was not a nurse and so she was not given an emergency petrol ration and she was therefore unable to attend the appointment. The hospital phoned me. Did *I* still wish to attend? You bet I did! I had already had one setback. Between us, I myself, the breast care nurse and my husband would do what we could.

And so we did. I wish I could say that the session left me feeling good, but, despite everybody's efforts, that wasn't really the case. The specialist had rung in her advice to help us. Normally, she advised, a lady who has lost a left breast would wear a left breast prosthesis – logical – but *in my case* (oh, here we go again) it would be a good idea to try right breasts on my left side to give the right degree of fullness in appropriate places. Well, we tried and we tried. The simple truth was that breast forms which were big enough to match my remaining 'G' cup right breast were all too wide for my 34" ribcage, and so overlapped the remaining breast when I put them into my bra. It was so frustrating to feel, yet again, a freak. (Thank God for my brother, who when I recounted this to him said, 'You are not a freak; God simply made you unique,' and he somehow made it sound special.) Anyhow, we were on the point of giving up when my husband suggested that I turn the breast form through ninety degrees and try wearing it sideways, thereby making it narrower.

Initially, I snorted in derision, but was persuaded to try and the result was actually not bad. I dressed and looked in the mirror and I looked pretty normal. The nurse said she thought I looked 'pretty good' and it was certainly the best I'd looked all day, so we agreed I'd take that breast home for a trial run. The fitting with the specialist was rescheduled but if I decided later that I didn't need it, I could cancel.

I suppose I should have been happy, but I was close to tears on the way home. My husband asked why and I explained that it was no joy to once again feel abnormal. He said, 'I don't understand. I thought you'd be happy that they've given you something that makes you look good.' Now I bit! 'Suppose,' I said, 'that you lost your left leg in a car crash. Suppose you waited for the stump to heal and then went to be fitted with a prosthetic leg. Suppose they said to you, 'Well, normally we'd fit you with a left leg, but we don't have one like yours, so we'd like you to wear a right one and we'd like you to wear it sideways.' How would *you* feel?' While he didn't entirely accept the analogy, he saw the point!

I didn't get on too well with that breast, either. Being worn sideways, it tended to tilt at an angle in wear, and the bottom seam tended to roll into my skin. Within two days, I had what seemed to be an allergic histamine skin rash, or maybe a sweat rash, and from that point on, I had to wrap the wretched thing in a clean handkerchief before putting it into my bra. Also, I'd been given two silicon shoulder defenders to prevent my bra straps from marking my shoulders with the weight of my breasts (something I'd always lived with). These too provoked a reaction and stripped the skin. I wound up with two large blisters on my right shoulder that lasted a week. I was actually glad to have a bona-fide excuse to stop wearing those things; at least there were two less bits of myself to assemble every morning. I had begun to feel like the lady in the old music-hall song!

In time, I duly attended the rescheduled appointment and the specialist found me a better solution. It was still a right breast, but this one, being more of a tear drop shape, sat better on my chest. Apparently it was an old model – one that the firm had threatened to discontinue, but it suited my need, and they gave me two cotton covers for it so that I wouldn't have any more uncomfortable reactions. It moved around a lot less, and I was much more comfortable with it. And wasn't I glad now that I hadn't opted for any instant reconstruction with silicon after all those possibly allergic skin reactions! Imagine something like that happening on my *insides*!

About the whole business of breast prostheses: inevitably, since the woman concerned has lost a breast, a precious part of herself, she needs to find something very like that missing part in order to restore her confidence. Although the silicone shapes on offer are a very good attempt, and although those who fit women with them have endless patience, there is, it seems to me, still some way to go. Some prostheses rejoice in names like 'nearly me' and, for some customers, they truly are. I, on the other hand, wanted to replace such legends with heavily loaded phrases: 'in your dreams', 'no earthly comparison' etc. for I did not feel that such pieces of uncompromising synthesised fake flesh could make me feel whole again. I was, of course, expecting too much; God had created my original body, and man and plastics were no substitute, but wouldn't anyone in my circumstances have had similar expectations? The best that could be said was that once fully clothed in a garment with a suitable neckline, the prosthesis in situ looked just fine and felt very natural. It really did. For many women, this is quite enough. Ladies I know well have chosen this path and truly look great. Maybe I was ungrateful, but I wanted to be *me* again. Every person's journey is unique…

So the treatment proceeded and I did in due course have my second bout of chemotherapy. For each person on such a regime, the pattern is slightly different, because our reactions to the various drugs are individual. For me there were three to four 'alien' days, followed by another when I would feel slightly nauseous. There would also be three or four days of acute bone-centred pain in the back of my skull, radiating down the back of my neck and across my shoulder blades. This caused me great anxiety at one point, because, when I telephoned the chemotherapy nurse to discuss it, I thought she would say something reassuring like, 'Oh, yes, that's just part of the chemo.' That very reassurance was, of course, what I was looking for. However, she said she felt I should have an oncology appointment within the next few days to discuss it with the doctor, who might order some tests… 'Such as bone scans?' I asked, and I was now *really* scared. She responded, 'If he thinks they're necessary.' I didn't want anyone looking to find any more cancer in my body at this point. I already had all I felt I could deal with. Logically, I can see now that if I reported a symptom it had to be investigated, since I may otherwise have demanded later to know why it was not, but, at the time, the thought of finding anything new to come to terms with scared me half to death. In the event, the oncologist simply examined my chest with a stethoscope and pronounced that the bone pain was likely to be a reaction to the withdrawal of the steroids, which are only taken for four days after each chemo session. I would have spared myself so much angst if I had stopped to listen to the inner voice telling me, 'Fear not…'

After the bone-pain phase I experienced a roughening of the lining of the mouth. Some patients develop ulcers at this point. Of course, it isn't just the lining of the mouth which is stripping, but, to some degree, the entire alimentary canal, as I discovered to my cost when I ate a good chilli one night just as this process was beginning… This phase, for me, lasted four or five days initially. As the chemo cycles progressed, it seemed this stage in the process became more marked. I was often queasy, and that queasiness often persisted far longer in later cycles.

Tiredness and aching also seem to be 'par for the course'. I sometimes felt very easily moved to tears and seemed emotionally very fragile. I cried an awful lot. The weakness was hard to bear as I felt that I had been suddenly catapulted into my nineties, struggling when I wished to rise from a chair or my bed. Sometimes, I had to roll from the sofa onto my knees on the carpet and haul my way up. I could no longer take the regular evening strolls with my husband. Instead, when I was up to it, he would accompany me round the block. I began to feel I would go stir crazy.

Another side effect which caused me considerable embarrassment and inconvenience was flatulence. This may have been partly due to my change of diet, but I am sure, having conferred with other patients, that it is also a part and parcel of the chemotherapy process. One can only, as one of my friends also undergoing treatment pointed out, say, 'Pardon me,' so many times in any one day, and the whole business became not just irritating but humiliating, although my family members were very good about reassuring me that there is no point in getting upset about something you cannot help, and over which you have little or no control. At least this experience kept me firmly grounded in my humanity!

I discovered also that one side effect can be vivid and graphic nightmares caused by the effects of the drugs upon brain chemistry. I frequently had strange dreams during treatment, but only one really dreadful nightmare. At the time it was very, very vivid and spilled over into my waking hours, but I would not share its content with anyone because I didn't want another person to be left with the mental images I was carrying. Now, mercifully, I can barely recall it. However, it was just one more thing to have to put up with among the many – and chemotherapy is cumulative, so the symptoms can tend to become more severe the further a person is into the process. The support and understanding of family and friends is crucial, and I was blessed with a very good support network. I didn't, for example, feel able to drive with any confidence for a while after each chemo session, or on 'tired' days, as I felt I would be a threat to the safety of others. My friends rallied round in an amazing way, and I seldom had to get behind the wheel unless I felt ready to.

The expected gynaecology appointment came through, and the prospective surgery date was to be the Monday before my third chemo session, which would take place on the Thursday. The oncologist was happy with that, so I attended a pre-admission clinic and all was set up. It was proposed that the surgeon would perform a laparoscopy, just to have a good look inside the whole pelvic area, a hysteroscopy to have a good look inside the womb, a D and C, (dilatation and curettage) to clean out the womb lining and anything else of a minor nature considered necessary. In the event, he removed a couple of polyps as well. However, there was so much more…

I had talked at length to a friendly priest about the whole question of a possible pregnancy and its prevention in my present circumstances – and he was the second priest I had consulted. The first had counselled that, in these particular circumstances, whatever we decided to do was right and he was not going to interfere any further, although he did say that he felt that total abstinence from sexual intercourse was not an advisable option and that abortion would be the worst of all possible outcomes – but this last was something we had already decided we could never countenance. The second priest said that, in our case, he felt that sterilisation was *advised*. He said that this was not a suggestion he made lightly – indeed he had only ever given such counsel once before – but he felt that in this instance it was a decision both medically and morally justified. He also said that he felt that the preservation of our close and loving emotional and physical relationship as a couple was paramount.

Now, I had spent a great deal of my life during the early part of our marriage on fertility treatment…had conceived at least three times…had never carried a pregnancy to term and had never, until now, had to think about preventing one. What was more, I had always felt that the hormonal changes of the menopause might have given us one last chance to add to our family, since the prolactin that helped to render me infertile by being present at too high a level in my body (usually produced in this quantity only in the bodies of nursing mothers) might have dropped at this time and given us a chance to conceive. This last chance began to look less and less likely. Though the oncologist said he didn't believe that I was going to conceive whilst on the chemo, he couldn't say it wouldn't happen. Though people taking Tamoxifen to aid in conception do not take it every day as I was doing, we could not be sure that it wouldn't make conception more likely. Though American research, as I have said, appeared to have shown that some babies conceived on chemo come successfully to term, I believed the study was small. And, in addition to all of this, I was on the Tamoxifen in any case to attempt to suppress the very hormones any pregnancy would promote, because any cancer cells still remaining in my body would feed off them, grow, and make me ever sicker, perhaps even unto death... Thus, even though the oncologist felt that I would be *unlikely* to conceive (but it was *not impossible*) and sterilisation was not, in his view, necessary, my priest counselled that sterilisation was the least of the evils facing us – if I could face it without feeling that yet another aspect of my femininity had been taken from me... I was only certain that I could never kill my unborn child; NEVER, not under *any* circumstances...

The morning of the surgery arrived and I finally met with my surgeon. He reviewed my notes, particularly the query over possible sterilisation, and counselled very strongly in its favour on medical grounds, arguing that it was never going to be safe for my body to experience the hormones of pregnancy again, (though of course it would be possible for these hormones to be set in motion as long as I was fertile, and at this point no-one could be sure when that would cease). I knew what my spiritual advisers had said, but this situation was still so hard for me to face. On this very morning, I asked God for a sign. I had a second visit from the gynaecology consultant, still strongly recommending sterilisation as the appropriate medical decision, and a visit from my close friend, the midwife, who has shared my spiritual journey for many years, and who also felt that sterilisation was the right course of action in the circumstances. And so, with my husband at my side, also convinced of the rightness of this course of action, I gave my consent. I had done my best to take advice both medical and spiritual, and I had to make a decision. If the procedure was to take place, the only logical time was now, when I would be cut for other reasons and therefore ready. I had my surgery.

I was completely unprepared for the way that I would feel after the event. I had had no idea that I would become so *very* distressed. Initially I thought along the lines of, 'Oh well, at least a decision has been made,' and that was a relief, but I had never thought I would have to face up to sterilisation, as it was something that I had always felt would be wrong, going against my conscience and perception of God's will for me, yet, backed by the advice of God's appointed ministers, I had done it. I knew that I had taken all possible steps to ensure that I was doing the right thing and acting in good conscience, but now, unaccountably, I felt 'different'. I had the strangest feeling that I had somehow 'sidelined' myself with God and had blocked one channel through which He worked in my life. He had been answering a lot of my recent prayers and I had been conscious of great blessing. Now I feared, irrationally, that might cease. I cried so much, both day and night, and I endlessly questioned the decision I had taken. I was seriously at risk of giving way to depression, which can, in itself, be a side-effect of chemotherapy. Thankfully, help was at hand.

Christian friends were alarmed at my response. One pointed out that the power of evil does not play fair; Satan loves to attack you when you are weak. – And what better way to attack than to convince you that you have somehow become distant from God? Another friend received a word from the Lord when she was praying for me. She did not tell me immediately, wanting to be sure that this message *was* from God and not simply a product of her own desire to help, but over a time she became very sure that this word should be passed on to me, and something that I said to her one day in the course of a phone-call convicted her that this was the time.

She told me that the Lord would have protected me from pregnancy in any case, but that He had known that I would not be able to relax without the added security of the sterilisation and therefore He had allowed me to be free and to make that decision, aware that no amount of 'words' or scripture readings would have convinced me that I was really safe. She said that He was distressed to see that I was now so upset – for the decision that I had taken had not affected His plan for my life. It was not part of that plan for me to actually bear children. There was more, too, but of a more personal nature, and as I absorbed this and the wise counsel of other good Christian friends, I began to recover and to regain my sense of proportion. Also, I was to see in time that God was still very much answering my prayers for others in clear and dramatic ways.

I had been praying for two different families in my parish where relationships had become very strained and healing of rifts was much needed. Over the Christmas period, as I was coming to the end of my chemotherapy, I heard real evidence that things were improving in both families. Delighted at this, I also rejoiced for myself, for I felt that God was showing me that He still loved me, still heard my prayers, indeed wanted to show me the great **depth** of His love, wishing that I understood how much He cared.

Now I believe I have come to terms with what was essentially a medically necessary decision but it took quite a while. Our parish priest told my husband that he thought I would not be happy until I had polled an entire bus queue and found someone who would tell me I had been wrong! He himself stated that the decision was clearly medically justified.

Looking back, I can see that I was very weak at the time that I was so troubled. No one would suggest that four lots of surgery, chemotherapy, and heart-rending, serious decisions are good bedfellows, yet I had been struggling to cope with the lot! I cannot speak highly enough of what God did for me during my chemotherapy treatment, for I was far less sick than I might have expected to be, and the side effects that I experienced were limited in their severity. Yes, I was nauseous, yes, I was weak. I was also subject to mood swings and found it very difficult to stay positive all the time. Indeed, for much of the period that I was under treatment, I battled inwardly against myself. Everyone said that I had to remain positive – that I had to believe that I would get well – but I didn't see how I could state that as a certainty. After all, don't Christians pray every day, 'Thy will be done'? If we mean what we pray, then surely we have to accept that the will of God might not be in accordance with our current desires. I felt certain that God would make me well as long as that would be for my ultimate good, but I am not God. I cannot see the whole picture as He can. People told me over and over to 'be positive' and inside myself I struggled for true abandonment to the will of God. I know that haven't, even at the time of writing, totally achieved that, though I regularly reaffirm my intention of surrender. I know that God's will for me is for my ultimate good. I know that there is no point in trying to keep part of my life under my own control, for to believe that we ever *have* control in our uncertain world is just a delusion. Many years ago a road traffic accident in which our son was injured taught me that! Free will we have, but control over our lives in events where others are involved we do not. Only when I can give my life completely to God will I be sure that I have nothing to fear, for everything that He allows to happen to me will be for my good, yet at this time, when I tried to pray a prayer of total abandonment, I found a part of me wanted to hold something back.

If what I have just said sounds odd to you, then think for a minute of the things in your life that you hold most dear. What if abandoning yourself to God's will meant that you would have to give up the very thing that meant the most to you? Even if it was for your own good, could you do it? This, of course, is where trust comes in. I am slowly learning that we often imagine that God will act in a certain way without considering His great love for us. He is unlikely to ask us to relinquish those gifts that He has given us that we hold most dear, but sometimes He has to, only because greater good for us will be brought about if we do. Sometimes it is very hard to see how the loss we incur can possibly be for our good, but perhaps that is because our sight is so limited, so blinkered, and His is so broad, spanning space, time, eternity. Through this experience of sickness I was gradually learning about trust, and greater gifts of faith and trust would certainly make my life more secure and less anxious. Perhaps, in the end, this will prove to be what it was all about. I just hope and pray to move closer to Him, so that each time, when I say I have given my life to Him, there will be a new meaning and a greater depth in that statement. After all, as the disciple said, where else would we go? For each of us, our walk with the Lord is a lifetime's experience, and there are lessons everywhere. I learned a lot through this first year of treatment, but God has by no means finished with me yet.

Thankfully, I was able to attend church throughout the treatment and this meant a great deal to me both socially and spiritually. I was not able to mix normally with others, either socially or in the workplace, because I was so at risk of infection.

I could not attend parties, for I did not know what potential risk factors those present might be carrying, nor could I go to the theatre or cinema, because someone who was coughing or sneezing might have come to sit close to me, and I would have been trapped. I could not go in to work, though I tried on numerous occasions, because the chemo nurses, when contacted for advice, felt that I would be at far too great a risk of infection from contact with the children in the school. Church, however, was different because, from the very beginning of the treatment and throughout, I had been part of this 'germ pool', regularly seeing the same people. What is more, they knew that I was at risk and always took steps to protect me. I had to keep my distance from those with colds or coughs, and often I had to sit when others stood or knelt. Sometimes I felt rather strange or suffered hot flushes, but I went to church every Sunday and on most occasions when I was due to play guitar, I did so. I also frequently attended my usual prayer groups. On one occasion, playing at the London prayer meeting, I was unable to stand as I usually did to play, during the second half, when the prayer for healing is offered, so I sat – and was touched to find that the two big fellows between whom I was playing on that particular occasion also sat, without a word, in order to keep me company and that I might not look odd. Such solidarity!

During the run-up to Christmas and during the latter half of my chemotherapy, the mixed denomination drama group at church was working on a production for Advent, a variation on the traditional nativity play. Many in this group were close and had been in regular contact since the onset of my illness. They asked me to take part, making it very clear that they understood that I could not always be reliable and telling me that they would fully understand if I was not, as it were, 'alright on the night'. Knowing that it would mean only one weekly rehearsal, (if I was up to it) and very keen for any activity that added spice to my somewhat slow pattern of living at the time, I said that I would enjoy taking part, and agreed to be part of the chorus.

I had to miss some rehearsals. Also, I sometimes had to sit alone in one block of pews in the church while everyone else sat in another, so at risk of infection was I! They laughingly tolerated my lone voice from the left, and even my irascibility and evident tiredness. When the time came to rehearse on stage, I was allowed to sit out if I needed to, and during the performances, I was to be always positioned in front of a pillar, for strategic leaning! How incredibly kind and accommodating they all were, and what a sense of achievement I had from being included. They protected me utterly, from start to finish, guarding me from fevers, flu and over-exertion, ferrying me back and forth, and encouraging me when I was low.

I did, by God's grace, get through it, though I had arranged a stand-in for everything I had to do or say that mattered, just in case. I did a lot of leaning against that pillar, and I felt sometimes weak, sometimes lousy, sometimes weepy, but they were there for me, and being a part of that nativity, even for an hour or so each week, made up for the fact that I was missing the seasonal choral events in school that I have always so much enjoyed being a part of. I just couldn't risk going into school at a time when half the pupils, and, it seemed, all of the staff, were coughing and sneezing, so I missed all of the festivities there, even the concert, for how could I be seated in isolation in an assembly hall?

When it was all over, the nativity cast gave me a potted plant and a card that read as follows:

'The order of the Christmas Cactus [second class] is awarded to Helen Gaize in recognition of the fact that she, despite numerous assaults on her person by various members of the medical profession, [such attacks included, among other things, stabbing her repeatedly with sharp instruments and uttering loud cries of 'One Hundred and Eighty' whenever they managed to draw blood] was a regular attendee at rehearsals at times when she would much rather have been tucked up in bed.'

Of course, over that period of time, those people had given me far more than I ever gave to any of them, and I shall always be grateful.

The references to 'stabbing... with sharp instruments' were more than valid. In the course of the treatment, my difficult veins became impossible. There were two particularly memorable occasions. The first was when the treatment line was actually safely sited within my vein, but the flow of the drug (Epirubicin on this occasion) was obviously sluggish. The nurse investigated with a saline 'push' (a syringe full of saline pushed into the line to see if it flowed properly into the vein) and it became evident that the flow into the vein had stopped and a small amount of the drug had pooled in my tissues. This caused great concern, as it is a cytotoxic drug, harmful if it goes into the tissues rather than the circulating blood. I was sent out of the treatment room with an ice-pack on my arm and had to elevate it for forty-five minutes. The arm was thoroughly examined by doctors and it was pronounced that a plastic surgeon would not be needed. What a relief! However, the wrist area, where the leakage had occurred, remained very swollen and painful for months.

On the second particularly memorable occasion, my chemo appointment was for ten o'clock that morning. I was actually called in at half-past, but by twelve o'clock, though they had tried five times (and wiggled the needle about in my arm on each occasion) no one present had managed successfully to get a line in. It had been painful trying, to say the least, and by the time they did manage and the treatment could start, I was tearful and past coping. At the best of times, who wants these alien substances in their veins anyway? On this, one of the more gruelling occasions, the prospect of the forthcoming side effects was hard to bear…

Despite the problems I have mentioned, my chemotherapy came to a successful close four days before Christmas, praise God for such timing! It had been April when I had noted the abnormalities in my breast for the first time, and looking back I felt I had been walking a long road. I saw the oncologist after the final treatment and he congratulated me, then he reminded me that any treatment I had received since my surgery, and any I would receive from this point onwards in radiotherapy, was precautionary. It had not been planned because I was sick, but to prevent further sickness. I was not, therefore, to be looking over my shoulder for the disease to return, for this in itself would raise my stress levels and weaken my immunity.

Christmas itself was a quiet affair of only immediate family and the friends associated with church, because it was felt that it would be dangerous for me to travel to meet with the extended family or to attend any parties, lest I catch influenza or some similar winter illness. I coped fine with Midnight Mass and thoroughly enjoyed being involved with the music – the grace and blessings that made this possible were my Christmas gift. The Midnight Masses at Christmas and Easter have always seemed particularly special to me. To have had to miss out would have been awful.

Christmas dinner meant a morning of juggling in the kitchen in order to ensure that everything for a proper meal was ready on time. For the sake of the children, we were determined that none of the important ingredients must be missing, and, where necessary, I provided alternative menus in order to meet the requirements of my diet as well as everything my children would expect. I orchestrated many of the preparations from a sitting position at the kitchen table, and there, too, I peeled the outer leaves from the sprouts. The family members scuttled about willingly enough at my bidding, since none had ever organised such a dinner from start to finish before.

It all came together perfectly on time and we thoroughly enjoyed ourselves, but by the early evening of Christmas Day I was truly past it; it had only been four days since my final chemo treatment and I was still very fragile. At one point, I walked into the lounge and my husband and son were watching 'Titanic'. They were just at the point where death and destruction are everywhere. I watched for a few minutes and then dissolved into tears: 'I can't do this today,' I sobbed, and left the room. They came quickly to find me and told me to return. In empathy and understanding they had switched it off. We spent a cosy Christmas evening with board games and I was not late to bed.

In the same vein the days passed gently until New Year, which we celebrated once more with games – cards this time; there has to be some variety! – on New Year's Eve, followed by telephone calls to the family we could not join for fear I would succumb to infection, and calls also to family members in New Zealand. At the best of times I find it hard to get the 'time thing' right, but in the state I was in then, it was hopeless. My sister actually expressed a belief that I might be slightly drunk – not so, for I had only had half a standard glass of wine, but I must have sounded less than with it over the phone!

I was expecting my radiotherapy to begin in January. This was one of the things that the oncologist had mentioned when I had seen him after my final chemo treatment and he had been so very positive, reminding me on that day that all the treatment that I had received since my surgery had been precautionary – 'belts and braces stuff' – and that I had no reason to believe myself other than well now. I was, you will recall, to go forward optimistically, because, if I was constantly anxious, waiting for problems to appear and for the disease to return, then I would compromise my immune system and make that scenario more likely. I should move on to my radiotherapy, and then resume my life!

I had been marked up in readiness – twice! The first time I was asked to attend for this process had been in the middle of my chemotherapy course. I attended the nominated hospital in Cambridge, more than an hour's drive from my home. I presented myself at the correct reception point, and in due course I was collected by a smiling and helpful member of the radiotherapy team, who took me round to the simulator. This is a very clever piece of apparatus which uses fine beams of light from above to help to position the patient very accurately on the treatment bed, in order that, when radio-therapeutic beams are delivered, they target only the correct treatment area, and do so consistently. The bed itself is in fact a hard table. It has to be, because if the patient was progressively sinking into a soft bed during the treatment, the field receiving the treatment would be undergoing a constant change. The patient lies upon this table in order to have their body marked up to ensure accuracy of treatment.

For a breast patient, the table is first prepared by having the 'breast board' added to it. This is a board which angles the bed upwards towards the head end, so that the position of the patient will be as if reclining on pillows. The patient, once again naked from the waist up, then climbs onto the table and is requested to raise her arms and rest them in the stirrups behind her head. There is a solid ridge on the table beneath her bottom to prevent her slipping 'down the bed' and a plastic covered foam wedge is placed in the crook of her knees to keep her legs comfortable and still.

The first mark-up process that I went through took twenty-five minutes and I found it more than daunting, I confess. Nothing nasty was done to me, but the process was new and somewhat frightening and I was very, very uncomfortable, after a little while. The reason for this was the position of my arms. They were, as I have said, in stirrups above my head, and it seems that either the blood flow or the nerve arrangement or both, in my left arm, was damaged a little by the surgery I had undergone. My reason for reaching this conclusion is that it took very little time, once my arms were in the stirrups, for the left hand and arm to firstly tingle, then become numb, then begin to hurt, and hurt appreciably. The radiography team members were working around me constantly. Every now and again they would need to quell the lights, leaving me in semi-darkness in order to be able to see the red and green beams of light, used to mark my body, correctly. Often, they left me in the semi darkness to go into an adjacent room from which they took x-rays to ensure that the positioning of the machinery in relation to my body was correct. My arm was very uncomfortable and I was fearful of not being able to remain in the required position. At such times, it helped to chat to the Lord. We are blessed to know that we are never completely alone, even when in fearful circumstances in an empty, darkened room…

At the head end of the radiotherapy table is the apparatus that delivers the radiation as desired. On the simulator it is not treating the patient, but its exact position in relation to the patient's treatment fields is being worked out, to ensure *effective* treatment, so this cumbersome piece of machinery moves around, beside, behind and over the reclining patient. It can, at times, be a little claustrophobic, though the patient is never enclosed. When the apparatus is directly above the patient, a glass plate may be fitted below it, onto which 'leads' (like weights) may be put, so that these come between the beam and the patient's body and so will mask off areas that do not require treatment when the therapy is delivered. A template for each individual patient is drawn up, once the leads are correctly positioned, to ensure that they will always be in the same place during treatment.

Because this was my first time in such a situation, I really felt very anxious and insecure. Here I was, surgically mutilated and once more unclothed, among a team of busy total strangers. From time to time, I was alone in semi-darkness, unable to move, with mechanical noises going on around me, and my arm really hurting. It may sound melodramatic to say this now, but I can honestly say that, at the time, crucifixion came to mind, though at no time did any part of the *process* actually hurt at all, despite the fact that my left arm was by this time in a state of minor torture! (When all was finally over and they said, 'You can rest your arms down now,' I had to use the right arm to lift and place down the left, which had become a dead weight.) Part of my insecurity at this time came, I am sure, only because I did not know what to expect. Later, during the actual treatment, I was to grow much more familiar with it all, but at this point it was all rather intimidating...

Once the team members were happy with the positioning they had done, the oncologist was called in to check their work. He, too, was happy with it. I looked up, vulnerable, from that table, and saw a face I knew for the first time. I was, I later discovered, to receive radiation to four fields in all. One burst of treatment would enter under my left armpit, presumably through the area from which my lymph nodes had been removed. Another, directed from my right side, would enter the area of the scar on my left chest at an angle. A third would be beamed from directly above me, and a fourth would enter from behind. These last two were designed to treat the area bearing lymph nodes in my neck – the area that it would have been too risky to treat surgically. At the time when I was being marked up, I understood none of this, except that part of the treatment should be designed to catch those lymph nodes in the neck which the surgeon couldn't get.

Once the mark-up was complete, I was tattooed. That is a literal truth. So important is it to locate the fields for treatment accurately that the patient receives small but indelible marks, made by putting a blob of ink powder onto the patient's skin and scratching it in to create what appears to be a tiny blue-black mole. Four or five dots later, I was finished!

Though I was now processed ready for the radiotherapy, it couldn't begin, because, at the time when all this was done, I was still on chemo. Both chemo and radio therapies tend to hit the immune system so, unless it is necessary to a particular patient's individual treatment plan, they are not administered together. Therefore, although the therapist presented me with a treatment plan, the oncologist took charge of it to rearrange the dates for me so that the course would not begin until after the chemo was finished. This was why, on the day of my last chemo treatment, I was advised that my radiotherapy would start in January. I had already queried some aspects of the way my radiotherapy had been planned with my oncologist. From what had taken place when I was on the simulator, I was not certain that the neck area that he had specifically said he wanted included had been part of the marking process – neither was he, so he said he would check. In the event, I had put on weight in any case, and there was need to repeat the whole process to once again ensure accuracy in targeting the necessary fields. Once this was done, I had a bit of a shock – the therapy could not begin until February because there was a Christmas and New Year backlog to be dealt with first!

When I had been told, way back in the early days of chemo, that my second chemotherapy treatment could not be administered at the time I had anticipated because my blood wasn't up to it, I had confided to the sister on the breast unit where my surgery had previously taken place, that it distressed me so much because, 'It means another week bald and breast-less'. Now my hair was just beginning to return – I once more had a hairline – but the further surgery that I had been promised seemed to be moving to a more distant future as a result of this delay, as did any plans for returning to work. After nine months of eating, breathing and sleeping cancer, any delay is not easy to swallow, but swallow you must, so I went home to await the start date. During this time, my oncologist permitted me to go into school and share in light duties. I went in a few times and really enjoyed being there, but then a tummy bug epidemic hit the place, with the result that one tenth of the staff and student quota was off sick, so I was banned from such an unhealthy environment! Now I would have to wait until after my radiotherapy to return!

The treatment date came around soon enough, and by then I had accomplished a major achievement – I had abandoned the wig! Indoors, I had been reluctant to wear it for a while. I found it incompatible with hot flushes. And by now, I did have a downy covering on my head. I had been brave enough to go swimming (great exercise for the arms prior to radiotherapy) without my wig, and one Sunday, I 'bit the bullet'. My daughter had said she felt it was time. I rang a very good friend. 'Do you think I *have* to wear the wig to mass?' I asked her. She told me that I should feel free to do whatever made me comfortable, regardless of the reaction of anyone else. I trusted her counsel, but was still apprehensive, and so, with the wig as a furry passenger on the seat beside me, drove the car to church.

Once there, I asked the priest, whom I know well, if he thought it would be O.K. if I came to church as *me* that week. It was not that I thought that *he* would mind at all, but I was afraid of the responses of other people, who would undoubtedly notice, as I was to play guitar during mass. He boosted my confidence instantly. 'What's good enough for Sinead O'Connor's good enough for you!' he said. And that was it. One member of the congregation came and playfully shook my hand, saying, 'It is a great pleasure and a privilege to meet the sister of David Beckham.' Many people grinned, but no one objected at all.

After a few more days, I washed and styled my wigs and put them away. My goal had, in any case, been to have hair by the time we celebrated my father's eightieth birthday, which would be in early March. There was to be a big, family party, held at my step-sister's house, and my brother and sister from New Zealand were to be present, with his wife and her husband and family. I was eager to be there and to be wearing my own hair! **I made it!** Many people congratulated me on how well I looked and admired my new, short (very short! I have seen coconuts with more…) hairstyle.

But before the party came the actual radiotherapy treatment. Frankly, the treatment was less daunting than the journey! I had to travel daily to Cambridge, and the journey itself took more than an hour. Sometimes, the whole round trip could take *four* hours. Martin used three weeks of annual leave in order to drive me, because I had been warned that I would probably be tired. I am not sure, in fact, whether it is the treatment or the travelling that makes this so. In any case, I don't think that all that time in the car helped my back at all, and I didn't think to check the seat adjustment for optimal spinal support, because my mind was, understandably, on other things. I should add here that the firm that Martin works for was thoroughly understanding of the situation and he was able to accompany me to almost every hospital appointment, throughout my illness. This meant a great deal to me.

On the day of my first treatment, I was counselled about skin care over the treatment period. I was advised to use only 'Simple' soap, or a particular brand of baby soap. This is because they contain no perfuming agents. Perfuming agents are often aluminium based, and metals on the skin of the treatment fields are a no-no. I asked if I might use baby shampoo on my hair and was told I might do so sparingly and must rinse very thoroughly indeed afterwards, ensuring that none of it could remain on the areas of skin being treated, having run down in the shower. I was told not to use any deodorant. This was not a problem for me. I had given up deodorant whilst in hospital, and I have not used it since. Initially, afraid that I would smell, I showered twice daily, but after a while my skin became rather dry, so now I shower thoroughly once daily, and I have found that to be truly adequate – and no one else has complained! The radiotherapist also told me that, if I wished, I could use a light dusting of baby powder for freshness, but I chose not to do this, as I find any talc very drying and I did not feel it was necessary.

I personally was not counselled on the subject of clothing, though some of my friends were. I think the members of the team could see that I wore soft sports bras which were unlikely to irritate the skin. In any case, during the radiotherapy, I made a point of wearing freshly laundered clothes which had had no contact with perfumes or other such products, and for this period I did not wear neck chains, partly in case of metal deposits on my skin, however small (I was taking no chances) and partly because of the additional inconvenience when undressing and dressing.

We waited in a cheerful communal area, us radiotherapy patients, and we developed a rapid intimacy, since we were there every day and all in the same boat. The atmosphere was warm. We compared rates of hair growth, the states of our disease and treatments and we congratulated those who reached the ends of their courses. When it was my turn, I was asked to go around the corner to the single seat outside the treatment room and it was here that I was counselled, one-on-one, about personal hygiene products and skin care. Moreover, I was told that if I did develop a skin reaction which needed soothing, I might use E45 cream, but no other. However, my skin remained good throughout, and I never needed to do so.

Once I had been given the general advice, I was taken into the treatment room itself. This was very similar to the room in which I had lain on the table of the simulator. I was to lie as before, naked from the waist up, upon the table to which the breast board had been fitted. Once I was there, the radiography team (always two to four people) would make all manner of fine adjustments, using the beams of red and green light, as before, to help them, until they were satisfied that I was in exactly the correct position. During this time, the lights were dimmed, but, because they did not at this point need to take x-rays, I was not now left alone in the semi-darkened room. Indeed, the members of the team chatted to me constantly, though they sometimes asked me not to respond. (Apparently, I breathe very deeply when I speak, and this makes the field shift!) Once I was correctly positioned, the team members would turn up the lighting and leave the room, walking round the corner to an area adjacent to the reception point. From here, they could view me by video camera and monitor my treatment by computer. These machines would keep an accurate record of the treatments I received, for the oncologist and for quality control purposes.

Firstly then, once my tattoos had been located and I had been lined up, the business part of the machine was directed at an area in my lower left armpit. From here, the initial treatment was delivered, presumably into the area where my affected lymph nodes had been, mopping up any stray remaining cancer cells, as intended. Next, the gantry was swung over to my right side, where it was aligned, I think, with the inner edge of my surgery scar (the previous position having been at its outer edge). From here, it appeared to be treating most of the scar area. Following this, it was swung to a position above my face. (The team came in, between treatments, to make all of these adjustments, sometimes dimming the lights, but I was never left in the semi darkness alone during treatment.)

Once the machine was above my face, the glass plate I had seen on the simulator was added and then my template was carefully positioned upon it and the leads put into place to block some unwanted parts of the beam, protecting, for example, the edge of my jawbone. Only when all of this was completely accurately assembled was the third treatment delivered. After this, the machine was swung around behind me for the final burst. It is not possible for there to be anyone with the patient in the room, due to the radiation they would receive, but everything is done that can be done to make the patient comfortable and to reassure, and because my husband expressed interest in my treatment (he used to be a hospital engineer) he was allowed in one day to observe the setting up, then taken around with the team to watch the treatments delivered.

During treatments, I did again have some problems with discomfort in my left arm, but I learned that there were ways that I could position it in the stirrups at the start of the process to minimise this. I also found the sensation as I was lying there with the machine whirring to be very strange. It felt as if the treatment table was moving from side to side, and something about the whirring made my teeth vibrate. I tried closing my eyes, but this only increased the sensation of movement and that worried me, so I chatted with the Lord, since He didn't have to leave the room for fear of radiation!

I became quite anxious sometimes during treatment, fearing I may have moved, but I was reassured, and was told that, in any case, the treatment plan has a built in range of tolerance, because no one can lie perfectly still, however hard they try. I asked so many questions that one therapist said I would soon know as much as they did, but they answered all and set my fears at rest. I had fifteen days of treatment, excluding weekends, and they flew by. There was, however, one Thursday when I could not have treatment because the machine was being serviced. This servicing is very important because of the nature of the treatment and the need for perfect accuracy. Such equipment must be very regularly checked, and it is in constant use.

On this day, we decided that we needed to *do* something – and something totally unrelated to the treatment, at that – so we went to London, to the Victoria and Albert Museum. I hadn't been there since I was a child. We enjoyed this free day so much! I had packed sandwiches because of my organic, dairy-

free diet, and the understanding staff allowed us to eat our own
sandwiches in their cafeteria, despite signs cautioning people
not to do so. We walked around the museum for about three
hours, having been advised at the outset as to what we should
aim to see. (There are receptionists/guides at the entrance.) I
did, of course, have to make regular sit-down stops, and the
adventure was a good way of discovering just how much I could
and could not do. I did not have the staying power I thought I
had. Possibly, I was the only person to be surprised by this.

When my period of treatment came to an end, we gave the
radiotherapy team a small 'thank-you' gift and left for the final
time, with strict instructions to keep up the skin care routine
for a further ten days, and a cheerful, 'We don't want to see you
back here again!' I saw the oncologist towards the end of the
course, and he told me that there was no reason to suppose that
I would now be other than well. He listened patiently to my
thoughts and my queries at this juncture, looked at a couple of
moles I was concerned about (I have had to have a few removed
in the past) and discussed my return to work. Originally he
had suggested that I might be able to return to work about six
weeks after the radiotherapy finished, popping into school to do
a bit of light paperwork in the meantime if I felt up to it. Now
he recognised that I was eager to return earlier to my job and
arranged to see me one week later to discuss that.

The reason that it was so easy for the oncologist to see
me the following week was that I already had an appointment
booked at a clinic that he would be attending in another hospital
– at the breast clinic where my diagnosis had been made – but
it was in order to once again meet my surgeon and discuss the
way forward from here. Once I had done that, I would look in
on my oncologist. I duly attended my surgical appointment and
was told, as I expected, that nothing could be decided for six

weeks or so, in order to allow my body tissues to settle down after the radiotherapy. That was fine with me, but the next turn of events I found I was unprepared for, although the breast care nurse had told me long before that it was likely and that it 'didn't mean anything…'

I was to have some scans. I was told that forms were being sent to the hospital in my home town, requesting a chest x-ray and a liver scan. These, I was told, were just part of the normal procedure. I found it alarming, however, that the oncologist was pronouncing me fit to return to work (he even gave me a letter stating that I was 'free of disease') but the surgeon would not proceed further without checking. I know that he has to protect himself. I know that we live in a society where people sue medical establishments and staff more and more frequently, and I was repeatedly told on that day, by first a nurse, and then a breast care nurse, and then my oncologist, that this was all just routine stuff. I know also that it is a good thing to know what you're dealing with and to make sure that things are as secure as you believe them to be. Yet I *so* did not want, at this point, to even contemplate the possibility that I could have further problems, and it was obvious to me that, if they were scanning my body like this, there was at least a possibility that they thought my cancer could have metastasised and spread to other tissues. And if *they* were considering this possibility, then *I* could not escape considering it.

Things were made worse for me at home the following Saturday morning. I was eating breakfast, with some friends who had stayed the previous night, when the post arrived. There was an appointment from the Department of Nuclear Medicine for a radioactive bone scan! I felt I had received a body blow. I should have expected it, and the request must have appeared in my notes when the oncologist told me that all the tests ordered were just routine, but once this letter arrived, it was difficult to get the implications out of my mind. I had confided to the oncologist that I was now feeling fine, except for some backache, which I attributed at least in part to the journeys to and from Cambridge for radiotherapy. His response had been that there was nothing to worry about: '*I* get that,' he had said. Now the persistent back trouble began to seem ever more sinister in my mind – and, through no fault of her own, the breast care nurse didn't help.

I telephoned her, wishing to be further reassured that these tests were just procedure. She assured me that they were. She told me that, if I still had problems, which was very unlikely, then I would not be feeling well. 'Oh, well,' I said, 'that's fine, then, because the only thing wrong with me at the moment is backache.' She became silent for a second or two, and then said, 'When did your backache start?'... 'NO!' I thought, 'DON'T GO THERE!'... Though she went on to reassure me that my midwife friend was likely to be right in her conclusion that the trouble was muscular (she had recently been round to massage the affected area), she couldn't say for sure that this pain was not symptomatic of a problem... 'That would be wrong of me,' she said. The wait for those scans was sure going to be a long one...

That backache was very slow to resolve. In fact, I believe that a spate of vigorous gardening, including the shifting of some heavy stones, had seriously aggravated a back weakened by inactivity whilst I was under other treatment and abused by the daily radiotherapy journeys – but this is with hindsight; at the time, the constant presence of the pain really frightened me. Whilst waiting for the scans, I popped into work from time to time, but I had been advised by my oncologist to try to get a holiday of some kind before my official return to teaching. Martin and I had been offered the use of a country cottage by our very thoughtful neighbours. We had also been invited to spend time with a friend who lives by the sea and a cousin with a large house down south past Ringwood Forest, but at the very time when we needed to go away, Britain was in the throes of foot and mouth disease, and all kinds of travel restrictions were in force. Unable to be sure that we would be welcome if we travelled to far-flung rural retreats, we decided in the end to base ourselves for a few days in Birmingham at my father's house and travel out to do something different each day.

We wandered around the Museum and Art Gallery, drove into the surrounding countryside when weather permitted, and admired the local live steam railway (always a must for Martin; it never ceases to amaze me how many places we just happen to visit will have a conveniently positioned heritage steam station). We only had a very few days, but they were days of genuine 'time out' and therefore extremely therapeutic. Dad catered for us – very well indeed – but our time was our own (including a chance to be part of my New Zealand sister's birthday celebration, as she was then in England – Bonus!).

And all the time I had backache. I would wake up and think, 'Is it there?' The fear over what it might mean was a constant presence. Of the tests that the doctor ordered, the first was simply another chest x-ray, so I duly attended outpatients' and it was done. The second was the liver scan, for which I was sent an appointment and before which I had to fast for a while. After the scan (an ultrasound involving much jelly and a rolling sensor exploring my abdominal area) I said to the doctor, 'I suppose you can't tell me anything…' to which the kind man replied, 'No. Looks normal!' I was very grateful to him. At least that was one load off my mind.

In due course, I attended the appointment for the bone scan. I had been very apprehensive about this, partly because, when I had mentioned the backache to the breast care nurse she had said something like, 'I suppose the scans will resolve it.' By now I was back at work and my colleagues were once again my support gang and also eager for information. I told one of them that I would be afraid to ask anything of the radiographer, because I would be worried if information was not forthcoming – especially as the other doctor had been so kind in giving me hope after my liver scan.

I had a complicated day on the scan date, because the gynaecology specialist had decided that I needed another hysteroscopy – to be done on the same day. Accordingly, I reported first to radiology to be injected with a radioactive solution which would bond to my bones. I then walked through the hospital to wait outside the 'gynae' area for my hysteroscopy, but because I was now actually radioactive I had to wait on the corridor instead of in the waiting room, so as not to put others at risk. (Young children and pregnant and nursing mothers are considered vulnerable).

During the hysteroscopy the doctor was extremely kind. He allowed me to watch the proceedings on a television screen and explained everything that we saw in helpful detail, being particularly careful to reassure me that nothing that he saw was in the least alarming and giving me reasons why he was sure of that. The procedure, without anaesthetic, was a little painful, so, in case my concentration had been poor due to that, he took still photographs for my file, showing them to me once I was dressed and going over his explanations again. When I left him, I returned to radiology for my bones to be scanned.

Maybe it was because I was so apprehensive that I picked up such bad vibes. I tried to see the screen the radiographer was so intent upon. I *tried* to read her facial expressions or to interpret her body language. I *tried* to glean any clues and to fish for reassurance, but beyond telling me that it was a 'routine bone scan', (Is there such a thing? It didn't *feel* routine to me!) she was giving nothing at all away – and I convinced myself that this was because she saw something sinister. How did *I* know whether every patient had exactly the same scans and received the same reaction from her? Was I dreaming it, or was there some focus on my lumbar spine? I left that room in such a state that I left my jewellery behind and had to return to collect it.

I had been given a call-back appointment to see my surgeon after the scans, but the date for the bone scan had been later than anticipated, so I rang the breast care nurse to ask if I needed to cancel my due appointment, six days after the bone scan, and make one for the following week. 'Oh, no,' she said. 'You don't want to be waiting that long. Keep the original appointment and if the scan results are not back we'll get them to fax them through to us for you. Just ring us a day or two before to remind us to arrange that.'

I duly did. Then, on the eve of my appointment, a bombshell dropped. I had a phone call telling me not to come – my results were not available. To my shame I have now to admit that I rang the hospital and really let rip. Later I had to make another phone call, this time in order to apologise, but I had been so anxious, so geared up, telling myself that I only had to wait until this particular appointment…just three more days…two more days…one – and now they were telling me I would have to wait another week. Why? My scans had not been read, so the results were not available to be faxed. Why had they not been read? Because the person who was due to read them had been on holiday and no cover was available. I had no choice but to wait…And still, I had backache.

Eventually that appointment arrived. I was shown into an examination cubicle and the dear nurse who had herself had cancer (and in whom I had found such comfort before) said, 'Your bone scan isn't in your notes.' I didn't quite reach the ceiling, but I *was* dumbstruck. Seeing my face, she said, 'Hang on a minute.' She left Martin and myself alone in the cubicle for a little while, and then returned just to pop her head around the door and give a thumbs up. The trouble was that I didn't know whether that meant that she had obtained the results or that the results were good…

Eventually the surgeon entered the room and spent some time perusing my notes before saying, 'Chest x-ray normal, liver scan normal, bone scan normal.' I made him repeat himself twice. I don't think he understood how very anxious I had been. At least now I knew that, at this point, the disease had not progressed beyond my lymph nodes and metastasised into my body. As far as we knew, I really was healthy once more. Now I could wait for the backache to gradually resolve, for its origin must be muscular strain or other ordinary causes. Now further surgery could perhaps go ahead.

Before it did, I had a question I wanted to ask. A girl I had met in hospital and with whom I had had chemotherapy had also wanted her other breast removed as a precaution against the return of her cancer, but she had recently telephoned, knowing this was what I intended to do, to tell me that her surgeon had advised against it. She had been told that further surgery would weaken her and compromise her immunity; that she should not have it done, that she was more at risk of a cancer elsewhere in her body than in the other breast. She warned me that I might be told the same. Citing her as my example and my source, I

asked my surgeon his views. At first he became a little angry
and said, 'I cannot discuss another patient,' but I explained that
I didn't want him to; that I was only trying to tell him why I was
asking…that *she* had urged me to check: did he feel that further
surgery was advisable or not? He told me that everyone was
different but that he would consult with his chief, then he left
the room. When he came back it was to say that, yes, the surgery
would go ahead. The other breast would be removed.

We plan events in advance, and, even as people of faith, we like
to think we know what is on the agenda. That is never possible,
it seems to me, in the scenario of breast cancer. I guess it is never
true in the life of any person who aims to give God the steering
wheel, either! One of my colleagues had travelled a similar route
to mine and had recently had reconstructive surgery, using her
own body tissues, at the hands of this hospital's surgical team.
I had seen the fantastic result, and my surgeon had promised
months ago to create for me 'two fried eggs' in place of my one
huge and one missing breast, using those same skills. Now he
stood in front of me and stated that yes, a team member had
done that for her, 'but I am not going to do that for you.' I
reminded him of his earlier offer to do just that. 'Yes, but since
then, I have been to another conference. We go to conferences
all the time. At this one, they told us that this technique is
seldom successful in tall women.'

He explained that my ribcage was wider and longer than
that of my colleague and consequently the roots of my breasts
were much larger. A surgeon would have to cover more ground
before beginning to build out, and I did not have sufficient body
tissue to allow for that. I would go through a painful and time-
consuming procedure for a marginal and unsatisfactory result.
This was the man who, some months ago, had **volunteered** to

make me two new breasts in place of the figure I had lost. I had asked him at the time how big they would be and he had said, 'A – cup, B – cup.' Now he was telling me this was absolutely impossible. In this field, surgeons are learning all the time. It was not his fault, but I had taken his earlier words to heart – had known where we were headed. Now I was once again at sea, and it wasn't fair. This was yet another example of 'in *your* case' wasn't it?

We talked some more. He told me that I could have small implants inserted to create the same effect. He said that I would have to think about whether I wanted those implants inserted at the time when he removed the other breast or at a later date. He himself felt that it would be better to wait. For now, the simple removal of the other breast was the best option. I was sent away, as I believed, to think about it, and told that my name would be added to the waiting list. Surgery could take place in as little as one month's time, but might be delayed much longer, even into next year, as it was considered non-urgent.

Later, when I rang the breast care nurse to discuss the implant option, I discovered that the surgeon had made the decision for me. He had put me on the waiting list for a simple second mastectomy and nothing more. I was going to have to settle for a flat chest for at least six months. I had been trying to make a decision about whether I could cope with waking up to discover that I had no breasts. I had been talking to friends and colleagues about my options. I had been reading up on implants. And all the time, I hadn't really had a choice at all. I think that my surgeon had felt that it would be unwise to stretch the skin over an implant, creating a larger surface area for the wound closure, when I had had an area of skin that had threatened to become necrotic with all the risks that carries, after my last mastectomy, but who knows?

I stood naked in front of the bedroom mirror and studied my battered body many times. I studied the whole side, then the flat side, screening off the whole breast and trying to imagine what I would be like. And I came to a pro-active decision. I would have to work at some body sculpting for myself. I would have to take some responsibility for improving the way my chest looked by working on my muscle structure. Maybe, if I did that, a flat, toned chest wouldn't be too bad.

I have briefly mentioned that by this time I had returned to teaching. My oncologist had allowed this return a full two weeks earlier than he had originally said he would, and I think that this was because, for someone who had been through what I had, I was in remarkably good health. I was still working very hard on my nutrition. I believe that God does not want us to turn such things into our religious practice, but He does want us to follow wise advice in order to help ourselves. We have all heard the story of the guy who prayed over and over about the wonderful things he'd be able to do for others if only God would let him win the lottery. Eventually, God said to him, 'O.K., O.K. Herb, but meet me halfway, eh? At least buy a ticket!' I felt that God had provided me, through the book I have already mentioned, and through thoughtful friends in my Christian fellowship, with much wise advice… with my 'ticket'. Whatever the reason, I was able to make an early return to my students, and had a letter stating that I was free of disease and might work part time on light duties. The writer of such a letter has obviously never worked in a school!

My headteacher was wonderful. He had employed a young man to cover for me and he told me that he would keep this man on in order that I might select which of my classes to focus upon and thus might build up to total fitness for the start of the new school year, rather than 'jumping off at the deep end'. This was a kind and sensible plan, and the presence of this young man in the classroom was a great help; he and I soon built up a comfortable working relationship of mutual liking and respect, and we shared a sense of humour – but where children are concerned there are always 'wild cards'. Essentially, my classes wanted *me*. Students would often make life difficult for my colleague when I was not around, so for the most part we settled for team teaching – I was not carrying the whole burden, but I was working full time, pretty much from the date of my return.

As a team, we worked very well together and the classroom atmosphere was mostly good. A few things which had morphed unhelpfully in my absence began to come back into line; I was grateful for the help of my colleague and he thanked me for my support in the classroom in matters of organisation and discipline, easier for me as I knew both the school and the children well. It would be difficult to express thanks enough for such an accommodating return to the workplace after a long illness; I suspect that such accommodation is very rare – and yet there is no denying that in the event it was a full-time and not a part-time return, and as such was, in many ways, very stressful. And I didn't necessarily do myself any great favours…

I have never really been any good at pacing myself. Right at the beginning of my return to work, I was already involved in another project. I have written earlier of being sustained by my involvement in the production by our joint churches during the Christmas season. Now it was Easter, and the three performances of our Easter drama coincided with my first week back at work, yet I had to be part of it… It was, by now, so much a part of my life. I worked my first week back and finished it by participating in three performances of the musical 'I Will Be With You' at the joint church, and I made it through everything, so He certainly was! That hand of God was evident in another complication, too.

A special aunt of mine had been ill for some years. Close to death two years before, she had been granted a reprieve, I believe in response to prayer, but now her time had truly come, and her final suffering had been such that we had prayed to God for His call to come soon and He had mercifully taken her home. She had been an anchor for me during some difficult times in my teens and I had never forgotten her kindness, support, and 'open house' policy. I *so* wanted to be at her funeral – yet it was scheduled for my second day back at work. How could I even ask, after so long an absence? I made apologies tearfully to my aunt's family, with a heavy heart. Then a persistent little voice in my head began to say, 'What if you find out later that they would have let you go, if only you *had* asked?' I knew that I had to find out, but I felt I was really pushing the limits. After all, I had been off sick for more than eight months. Tentative, I confided my problem to a senior mistress and asked if I should approach the Head. There and then, she herself wrote the funeral into the diary and told me that of course I must go.

When I finally arrived at the porch of the Birmingham church where the service was to be held, one of my cousins (all of whom have always seemed in my heart to be siblings, rather than cousins, so closely did we grow up together) clung to me, as I did to her. All she said was, 'You came.' That said it all for both of us. We have always had a special rapport, and I belonged there, at her side. It was a beautiful funeral and valuable family time. Living at such a hectic pace, we do not frequently enough consolidate our roots, yet particularly at times of flux and crisis we really need to be grounded and to be with the people God placed us among. They are in many ways our greatest stay in all things.

I had been following a Christian course at a very special place called 'The House of Prayer' at Abbotswick, near Brentwood. This involved attendance at a series of Thursday evening talks and exercises. It was led by a wonderful man, John Vaughan-Neil, and was called 'Sons and Daughters of the Living God'. I found the entire course very helpful, as did others. It was wildly over-subscribed. An important part of it involved a whole-day programme on a Sunday. During the day we would have opportunities for the Sacrament of Reconciliation (confession) and to attend Mass. We all took picnic lunches with us.

Because I am so aware these days of the importance of good nutrition, I pack my picnic lunches with care! On this particular day, I had made a huge and perfect organic, pink grapefruit the centre of my repast. (There has been some more recent research suggesting grapefruit is not helpful in breast cancer, but at the time, this was not known.) Imagine, then: It is lunchtime. I am sitting under a tree. I begin to peel my grapefruit and I see that there is a small maggot on the peel, which I presume to have come from the tree. I brush it off and finish peeling the fruit, which is without blemish. And as I prise it apart, I find – *seething maggots*. YUK! At the time, I am extremely annoyed, for this fruit which I must now consign to the bin was a substantial part of my lunch, but God is good, and a friend at my table says 'Would anyone like some grapes? There are far more here than I can eat!' and I am not slow to respond in the affirmative! At the time, that was that. An annoying distraction in an otherwise very good day...

Later, we had celebrated Mass and there was a quiet time before people went to receive individual prayer ministry.

As I sat in the silence, I had a stunning revelation and I understood my lesson of lunchtime. I had been reluctant, unable, as I have previously described, to give **everything** to God. There were bits I was loth to let go. I had been afraid that if I gave every aspect of my life to Him, he might ask me to give up my music – or to die of my cancer – and these possibilities had been just too painful to contemplate. Now, in the silence, I realised that I had been following an erroneous thought pattern: this part of my life I have given to God, this part of my life belongs in the realm of Satan (hopefully nothing at all in *that* box!) and this part I keep for myself, under **my** control.

Now it hit me like a brick. This was such a wrong way to think! Anything in my life that was not given to God belonged in the realm of Satan. There were no half measures! And **I was** the grapefruit. Everything seemed just perfect on the outside (there had been no external indication at all of either the maggots or their mode of entry) but there were nasties inside, destroying what should have been so good and with my tacit approval. I knew then and there that I had to give everything to God – and **trust** Him. Why should a God who has loved and sustained me so well for so long suddenly say, 'Aha! She finally decided to let go! Now we can do a thing or two that will really hurt!' The notion is absurd! God loves me. Anything that He permits to happen to me, He will use for my good. Satan is the one who wants me to believe that surrender to God will hurt me; and Satan is the Father of Lies. Oh boy, had I been listening to some! Joyfully, I was moving towards a new surrender, a new release, a more secure life in the Lord. I have since shared my 'maggots' story with many, and 'no maggots' has become a kind of maxim in my life.

So, I was working at school, and waiting for a summons for my surgery. When it came, I was given a date of June 22nd. I informed my superiors immediately. Around this time, I also bought myself underwear. At the back of my mind had been a constant fear that, for some reason, the surgery might not go ahead; maybe the cancer would return and prevent it; maybe the medical team would have second thoughts. And I so ***wanted*** this surgery, because, by now, I really craved symmetry. I simply wanted my body to be the same both sides. Sure, I was worried about the possibility of developing cancer in the right breast. Every time I showered, I looked down at it suspiciously. If, lathering myself, I thought I felt a lump, it was very worrying, because, when you have two breasts, the standard thing to do when you feel something in one of them is to check whether the other breast feels the same. Now I had lost my yardstick, and it is worth stating again that my breasts had always been prone to lumps. Cancer, therefore, was obviously a big part of the agenda, but symmetry was important too. Even before I had a surgery date, I bought crop-tops. My daughter and I reasoned that the sixteen pounds they cost was money well spent for the security of knowing that, if the surgery happened, I'd be set up, able to dress, afterwards. If it didn't happen, then perhaps a charity would benefit.

Once the date actually came through, I sorted out the things I would need for the stay in hospital. By now, I was something of an old hand and I began just by thinking about what I would need to do and to take. It is as well that I didn't get much further, because, with about a week to go, the nurse rang to say that my surgery had been postponed. I was, of course, non-urgent now, and a lady had been diagnosed in clinic and needed immediate surgery. Logically, and also by all that is right, no one could object to being postponed for such a reason. But when you are all 'psyched-up' and ready to go, neither logic nor all your Christian background prevents emotional turmoil! You hear your mouth muttering that you quite understand and you struggle to keep your thoughts under control, straining not to give way to a screaming rage! My friends from the prayer group had it right. They said, 'We must pray for the lady who needs your bed,' and we did.

I asked the ever tolerant breast care nurse whether I would have to go through the pre-op procedure again. In preparation for the surgery I had had a physical, had my blood pressure monitored, had an ECG to check out my heart, had a chest X-ray (yes, another!) and after all of these, I had had blood tests. The answer, when it came, was not particularly encouraging: 'not necessarily.' I asked whether, in view of the fact that I was non-urgent and had already been deferred once, this was likely to happen every time I got to the top of the list. The answer was, as you've probably guessed, 'not necessarily'. What else could the poor woman say? – But I have to say that, at the time, it was not particularly reassuring.

I was back on the waiting list, and at school I was heavily involved in my annual role as props mistress for the school production, a yearly, skilled and wonderful event involving literally hundreds of children. Last year, I had gathered many of the props, but because of the surgery had missed the great event (though on my return to school I found I had been rewarded for my efforts with quality real ale that was waiting in my pigeon-hole!) This year, I had not intended to do the job because I was convalescent, but two great friends of mine who had been for many years the driving force behind these professional productions, a husband and wife team, announced their intention to move on this Summer – to relocate. This would be their final fling. I had to be part of it. We had been a team for as long as I'd been at that school.

The play this year was a musical about evacuees, and I dutifully began making cardboard gas mask boxes for all members of the chorus, with the help of any colleague who would donate their labour. So many kindly did, thankfully. A second date came through for my surgery, this time in the second half of July, and I once again informed the world! At least this was right at the end of term, a few days after the production. Then one day my husband phoned me at work. Would I please, he asked, call the breast care nurses as a matter of urgency? I did. It was a Friday. Could I, they wished to know, come into hospital the following Wednesday, for surgery on Thursday? Wednesday was the opening night of the school play! Apparently, I should have received a letter, but the computer systems were down, so they were just checking that I'd been informed. I should have realised that the summons was likely to be soon, because the last time I'd attended the gynaecology clinic they hadn't had my records; they were being held on the ward. Of course, I said 'yes' and set about an orgy of last minute organisation. By now, colleagues just laughed when I gave them proposed dates!

Around this time, there was something else I had been trying very hard to organise, without success. The head, who had been so very good to me, and who had become a friend, was also leaving at the end of the summer term. He had decided to retire. I wanted to show my appreciation by buying him something special for his retirement. I knew he had a fondness for science fiction, having lent him some in the past, and I wanted him to have the C. S. Lewis 'Cosmic Trilogy', mainly because I had taken so much pleasure myself in these three books (Out of the

Silent Planet, Perelandra, That Hideous Strength), yet it seemed the novels were out of print in Britain. Worse still, my own copy of the three volumes in one paperback was missing. I had lent it out and forgotten to whom, and it had never been returned. The loss was a tragedy, because these works of fiction, so good to read and yet so gently informative about deep theological matters in true C.S. Lewis fashion, had been fond companions. I had recommended them to all and sundry. I confided all of this to the prayer group friends, half hoping one of them might declare that they had my copy, but no one knew where it was.

One kind friend, however, suggested trying to locate the book (or books) on the Internet, and this generous man worked at it for me for the next few days. He discovered that the work was in print in America, and showed me how I could buy it on line from there, but I was reluctant, as I now needed two copies (one to replace my own) and the postage and packing costs were prohibitive. Then we had a stroke of luck. He found it on a French mail-order site, and it was the American edition, in English. He does not speak French, but I do, and with his help and a little time, I navigated through the purchase process and the books were duly shipped to me, the postage costing only about three pounds. Result!

And it made me feel so good. Yet again, I had received help in need through a member of my ever patient extended family in Christ. There seemed no end to the ways in which they would put themselves out for me: transport, emotional support, little notes of encouragement, visits, flowers, cooking, the all important prayer, and now this last search. And then, by the grace of God, I had successfully made it through the French web site (my computer related skills, though pretty good now, were rudimentary at the time) which made me feel **such** a sense of achievement, both in terms of my I.T. skills and my French. Yes! I was high on the strength of the success of this enterprise for days! *And,* despite misgivings, the purchases arrived in time for me to give the boss his gift just before I went off for my surgery, and he was very well pleased. That was the icing on the cake.

As I said my farewells at work and prepared once more to go into hospital, I marvelled again at the goodness of colleagues. Teaching staff, administrative and office staff, cleaners and lunch time supervisors; all had nurtured me through this long process. I received regular little messages of encouragement, sometimes through the post, sometimes word of mouth, sometimes left on the doorstep. I could never thank the folks at work enough. Now, once again, their warmth encouraged me. I did my best to set my house in order and off I went.

I did not have to repeat all of the pre-op stuff; only the blood tests, and they were done the day I was admitted. I took my organic muesli and my golden linseeds with me and also my red clover, brewer's yeast, ACE and selenium and my noni juice ('What the hell is that?' seemed to be the general reaction). Noni is the juice of a fruit from a plant called *morinda citrifolia* which grows in the tropics. My window cleaner had recommended it to me and I had been intrigued and looked it up on the Internet. There I discovered that in experiments relating to lung cancer, it would appear to have been shown to be effective in fighting the disease, *not* by attacking the cancer, but by boosting the immunity of the patient. I took my findings to my oncologist who said, 'Yes, try it…It *may* help to boost your immunity.' I took it for a lengthy period of time: people I know of find it effective in a very wide range of disorders where a boost to the immune system can help. Of itself, it cures nothing, but with its help, people do get well. I firmly believe that during the whole period of my illness and recovery, God in His goodness made sure I found out about all sorts of things that could help me, and I am thankful.

On the day that I was admitted, I was visited by a surgeon. This, however, was not the man who had done my previous surgery, but the consultant who was the head of that clinic, and his boss. A learned and dedicated man, he has given me, and many other ladies, a new lease of life by means of his surgical skills. He asked to see my chest and I pulled up my nightshirt. He took a large black felt pen and drew two lines on my remaining breast. They were above and below the fullest part of my breast and marked out an area in the shape of a large eye that included my nipple. I asked him why he had drawn the marks there. I was alarmed, because the scar from my left breast mastectomy is a gentle curve *above* what was previously the site of my breast. I had always felt that my previous surgery was very neat (if perhaps somewhat thorough in terms of the amount of tissue removed) and had indeed told my usual surgeon so. If this man intended to cut where he had drawn, then, on this side, I would have a straight line in the **middle** of what had previously been the breast area.

I was desperate for the two sides of my chest area to match, as much as was humanly possible. I understood that a surgeon can never guarantee results because he is sculpting living tissue. Indeed, I think that in our search for eternal youth we often ask far too much (and frequently inappropriately) of medical science. Nevertheless, I felt the need to at least try for a similarity between the two sides of my chest. The surgeon plainly **was** drawing the line of his intended incision. We had a long conversation and I think I displeased him. I struggled to explain what I felt, and in the end I cried. He scribbled out the first line he had drawn and drew another, slightly higher, still using the same fat, black felt pen. My chest was now something to behold. I probably offended him, because I asked where my usual surgeon was. He responded, tongue in cheek, that he was away 'learning to be a proper surgeon'. Since both are extremely highly qualified, and respect each other greatly, and both go by 'Mr.' rather than 'Dr.', this dig at the other's reputation was amusing.

I know that the medic who was with me at that time is very academic and an excellent surgeon, and that he would never, at any time, do less than what he felt was his best, making wise decisions for good medical or surgical reasons, but I still found what he told me hard to accept. He said that the position of the original scar was, in a way, a mistake. It had been dictated by the position of the tumour. I said that I had thought that the incision had been made in that position because the scar from the original lumpectomy, which had been only partially healed when I went for the first mastectomy, had been vertical rather than horizontal. At this, he more or less said that proper mastectomies resulted in a horizontal line in the centre of the site of the original breast, implying that that was the only real way forward, then left me with my lines and the scribbling out on my chest, the fat, black graffiti feeling like an insult.

Later, another member of the surgical team, also a 'Mr.', also very skilled and dedicated, came to see me. He said 'You are going to end up with a line,' meaning that I would have the form of surgery that had first been sketched out. It was, he said, the only form of surgery that made sense. I spoke again of my desire for symmetry, and he said he would make the scar as high as possible. Then he, too, left. I understand from that visit that he was the one who was actually responsible for my surgery, but I have never been told.

The following day was a long one. I was last on the theatre list and it was an afternoon list so I did not go down until about four o'clock. All of us who were due for surgery had an early breakfast together, but after that there was little to do but wait. I watched beds wheeled down and back, saw the anaesthetist, received a pre-med in the form of suppositories (what fun) and waited.

Finally it was my turn. I was wheeled down and was met by members of the theatre staff, who were supremely kind. I did not feel the gloom and foreboding I had for the first mastectomy. Living with one very large breast had proved to be difficult and inconvenient. I had felt incongruous and had frankly rarely been able to feel sexually attractive, despite having a very loving and tolerant spouse. This had been mainly because, having to buy an H-cup bra for my remaining breast, and having been very limited in styles in order to properly accommodate this and the prosthesis, even if I kept my bra on when things became intimate, I felt I just didn't look the part. So much of sex is in the head; if you cannot feel attractive, how can you have any confidence at all? Having such a **huge** contrast between one side of my chest and the other, I just felt…well…*silly,* I suppose. At no time did my husband ever give the slightest indication that he found me any less appealing. I don't believe that he did. The problem was mine. I didn't feel sexy. I hoped that when my body was once more balanced, I would be able to live with it better and dress to feel more womanly once more – though I acknowledge that is a strange thing to say when contemplating the total removal of one's breasts!

Prior to the surgery, it was necessary once more to get some lines into my veins. Even before chemo this was always difficult. Now it was nigh-on impossible and eventually, despite my protests, they put one into my left hand. Ever since the removal of all of my lymph nodes from my left armpit, I have carried the card which states that this arm must not be used for blood tests, the taking of blood pressure…not for anything… Now the medical team was ignoring my protestations and shoving a line in, with an 'it will be alright'. I wasn't at all sure. However, they were good to me and the atmosphere, though professional, was relaxed and mildly jocular, and soon, in any case, I was asleep…

I woke in recovery and was surrounded once more by kind staff and medical paraphernalia. I had a drip line in my left arm and they were injecting a clear fluid into it – and it HURT! It really was very painful indeed, more painful than the surgery site. Apparently it was an intravenous antibiotic, Erythromycin, (I usually get Erythromycin as I am allergic to Penicillin) and it irritates the veins. I'll say it does! I don't know whether it was for general cover against infection, or whether it became necessary to give this because they were using the forbidden left arm, but it was the most painful part of this whole latest surgical experience. Once the drug was in and I just had the saline drip on that side, I was much more comfortable, though in fact that drip on the left never ran as it should and not long after I returned to the ward they removed it on those grounds, the nurse clearly expressing her displeasure that they had sited it there in the first place.

My first conscious action after the surgery was to put a hand up to feel my lower neckline; the area that you see in 'V' and scoop-neck clothes. Since the first mastectomy I had been rather self conscious, because the surgeon had, at that time, been quite aggressive about the amount even of fatty subcutaneous tissue he removed in order to be sure of removing all the cancer. He had removed breast, fat and muscular tissue, down to only a sparse covering of some remaining muscle over the bones of my ribs. I did not fully understand it at this time, but to all intents and purposes, most of my pectoral muscle had gone when the 'radical mastectomy' had been performed. There had been a line, mid-way in this neckline area, where the fatty layer on the right gave way to the skeletal area on the left. I had worked hard to improve the appearance of all this, and indeed my upper body in general, using weights (about one kilo) on a daily basis, with multiple repetitions of the exercises, each evening at home. It only took about twenty minutes, and I felt it was time well spent. Indeed, I had shown my chest to the breast care nurse and she had been impressed at the improvement of the wound site that had been so very hollow. It had certainly **begun** to smooth out nicely.

Encouraged by this, I had asked my G.P. to refer me to the local gym for a programme of exercise designed to fit my circumstances. He had done so and I had had an introduction to the gym and an induction to the exercises designed to meet my needs, but had got no further before I was called for surgery. However, I had hoped that this second surgery would smooth out some of the unevenness in the layer of fatty tissue and improve the appearance of my lower neckline. No such luck. Indeed, the whole right side of my chest, despite the mastectomy, was obviously a great deal higher than the left. No symmetry for me, then. This was a crushing blow.

In that post-operative situation and after all the careful consultation, I found this situation extremely difficult to accept. I was distraught, and the nurse, though patient, could not really console me. She said there had to be good, surgical reasons why the doctor had not, at that point, been able to make my chest area more symmetrical as I craved – that the surgeons were fundamentally good (I knew that) and would never deliberately make my life hard or do less than their best. (I knew that, too.)

However, once again I had a red slash in my chest, with two drain tubes, and as I looked at myself, I felt terrible.

In the centre of my neckline, I still had a point where the fat layer simply stopped, like a step. Living with this was odd; I found, for example, that if I wore a pendant necklace, there was a tendency for the pendant to turn over when it encountered this 'fall off'. They had simply not removed the subcutaneous fat on the site of the right breast as they had on the site of the left. This meant that, moving down from the neckline onto my chest, there was a prominent and appreciable thickness of fat remaining where the breast had been. It looked like a small breast; so much so that my midwife friend encouraged me to ask the doctor whether he had in fact removed all the breast tissue, or whether some remained. I couldn't believe it. I had made it very clear to the surgeons that I did not plan to wear any form of prosthesis after this surgery: why hadn't they given me a more even appearance? Why had they apparently not even **tried** to make me match?

Depressed, I waited for chances to ask the questions that filled my head. The answers came. Yes, all of the breast tissue had definitely been removed; what remained was simply fat. The fat had not been removed, because there is a greater tendency for the skin over the wound to become necrotic if it is. I was, they told me, a determined woman. I had vastly improved my left chest through exercise. That was to be my key now. The swelling on the surgery site would subside, and that would improve the symmetry a little. The fat deposit would lessen, because much of its blood supply had been taken away, and then I would have to work at body sculpting myself, building up muscle and whittling away fat through exercise in order to improve matters. Unhappy as I was, with that I had to be content.

The lady in the next bed was in a great deal of pain, due to a tumour in her back causing constant pressure on the spinal nerve. The nurses tried hard to alleviate this through medication, but they and the doctors knew that radiotherapy, which would shrink the tumour, was the only way the pain would really be stopped. There had been an attempt to mark Sue (as I will call her) up for her therapy, but, due to the pain, she had been unable to remain still for long enough. There would be another attempt later, once anaesthetists had been consulted. In the meantime, Sue had little real relief.

One night, she was obviously in serious trouble. I tentatively asked her if she had faith and she said, very positively, that she couldn't get through her days if she didn't talk to God. Would she mind, I asked her, if I prayed with her? Not at all. I left my bed, sat on hers, rested my arm on her shoulder, and prayed aloud. As I finished, I heard another lady in the ward, whose bed was opposite, say 'Amen.' This was totally unexpected and there was warmth and reassurance in the discovery, and indeed in the room. God brings the right people together at the right time; 'Where two or more are gathered in My name...'

Sue was visibly more relaxed after the prayer. She found renewed strength from this spiritual encouragement, and with God's help was able both to tolerate her mark up session and receive her treatment. Why don't we step out in faith more often? *I* had no means to help Sue, but through the grace of God she had been helped and being a tiny part of that was a blessing to all involved. I made a point of popping in to see Sue when I had occasion to visit the hospital for treatment after discharge, and once I went in just to take her some things she had asked for (and that was really my husband's initiative, not mine) and then, through my very human weakness, I allowed my visits gradually to decline. Returning from a week away, I rang one day to find out whether Sue had been moved, as she had expected to be, to another ward, and was sad to discover that she had in fact died, probably about a week and a half after my last visit...

Faced with news like that, I wondered if I could have done more: why hadn't I made a greater effort to be there for her? I felt I should have done. She had made her desire to see me plain. I knew how she valued my visits, yet I had allowed them to lapse and now it was too late. Yes, I have regrets but, as someone else once said, 'God uses cracked pots.' Even when we don't get it right. Maybe I need to learn to **listen** better, so that I can more clearly perceive and do the right or better thing, and that was the lesson to be drawn from this. Some lessons are painful. Maybe I was never meant to have further involvement. I am still not sure.

On this occasion my return home had been only four days after surgery (as soon as both drains had been removed) and as I had dressed in my outdoor clothes, ready to leave the hospital, I was apprehensive. I had been told by others in the ward that I looked like a schoolgirl in my short nightshirt and surgical socks, now that I had this smaller chest. The unevenness that bothered me so much was not greatly in evidence in my loose shirt and anyway the general consensus on the ward was that I had done the right thing in having the other breast removed, since I had appeared so very unbalanced. People felt that I looked better for the surgery. Even my daughter, who saw my naked chest, admitted that. Far from ideal it may have been, she agreed, but it was still much better than before.

Preparing to leave, I began to dress, donning one of my new crop tops instead of a bra. Prior to this I had not even been able to try it on, because the right breast had been too large for that to have been practical. I didn't even know if it would fit. However, despite the obvious difference between the two sides of my chest, the crop top looked O.K. and indeed went some way towards disguising the unevenness. I dressed in a lilac trouser suit – pants and tunic style – and I went home as soon as Martin was available to drive me.

I kept looking critically at myself. Martin made me turn slowly in front of him so that he could take in my new shape. He pronounced that, though I was different in left profile from right, both views worked. My shape was satisfactory. Well, maybe… but I was far from satisfied, and the situation seemed to worsen over the next few days. I became increasingly unhappy and anxious as a curious thing began to happen on the new surgery site. I began to feel that I had gone through the entire second mastectomy maybe for only a little improvement. I felt that my appearance was increasingly strange, for a woman who was now supposed to have no breasts. Each time I undressed, I looked at myself. It certainly appeared that I still had a small right breast, though without a nipple, and, alarmingly, it was still growing! Eventually, I said to Martin, 'This just can't be right. I'm going back to the ward.'

So about three days after my discharge from the hospital we returned in the middle of the morning to see a doctor. I have always appreciated the system at my local hospital that permits these walk-in visits. It is so reassuring to be able to have instant access to people that you trust when you are anxious or unwell. I saw a young female doctor that I had previously seen on the ward, and she was immediately both comforting and helpful. She took one look and told me, 'You've got a lot of fluid in there.'

So that was it! I had an explanation for my apparently growing 'breast'. Between my rib-cage and the layer of body fat they had left after removing the breast tissue, fluid was building up. Of course, at this point there was nothing connecting this fatty tissue to the muscles over my ribs, just a kind of pocket where the breast tissue had been, and this it was that had filled up with the fluid. The doctor now drained all of this fluid into a jug.

Both Martin and I watched in amazement as what seemed a huge quantity of pink liquid was sucked up by the large syringe inserted into my 'breast' and then discharged into the plastic measuring jug – several times. The right side of my chest visibly went down as if deflated. The doctor talked to me as she worked, reminding me of what I had been told on the ward; that I would have to exercise to improve my appearance. Because much of its blood supply had been removed, the fat deposit on the right side of my chest would tend to lessen, and I would work to build up muscle on the left side so that it would be less hollow.

In total, I had to have the site of my wound drained five times, usually about twice a week. Always there was relief after the procedure, but I wanted it all over and done with. They had told me that my best chance of long-term improvement lay with exercise and I wanted desperately to get started – but they wouldn't let me! I must wait, they said, until I ceased to need the wound draining and until six weeks after the surgery before I began to use the gym – and longer than that before I could resume the use of my weights. However, there was some good news on my last visit: we could take a holiday.

Almost immediately after I came out of hospital I had gone ruthlessly through my wardrobe. There had been surprises: some things that I had not particularly liked before and that I was sure I'd want to get rid of turned out to look quite good, while other things I loved and was sure would look O.K. just did not. Ah well! In the end I had a basic range of clothing and would just have to shop, really thoughtfully and carefully, to enhance that, so I didn't waste time! Who would, given an opportunity like that? Treats and a clear conscience! The sales were on, and my ever-thoughtful friends, knowing I would have this need, had given me vouchers for clothing shops for my birthday. I tried on almost everything in sight, for I had to learn how to dress to suit my shape all over again. In one shop the sales assistants watching my antics got the giggles, so I took them into my confidence about just *why* I needed to try on so very many garments and their attitude immediately became both sympathetic and helpful.

About one thing, I had been adamant from the start. As soon as possible after surgery I was going to visit the 'Nicola Jane' shop, a mastectomy specialist shop based near the South Coast. Martin took a day off from work (his bosses as always understanding and accommodating) and off we went. The long drive was worthwhile. I was desperate to buy swimwear and thought I should also buy a couple of bras, one black and one white, which would take small prostheses, for use when wearing clothes in which I couldn't really get away with my unevenly flat chest. I had thought I knew exactly which swimsuit I was going for, but trying on clothing is really important, and in the event, a different style from the one I had originally selected suited me much better. I bought two costumes in different colours but the same style. Neither had built-in prostheses, nor did I have to put any prostheses in; they looked fine as they were. What a relief that was! I could just get changed like everyone else, and no self-assembly involved.

I bought pretty lacy camisole bras in black and white, and tiny, minimalist, foam prostheses a bit like foam powder puffs, which could turn them effectively into padded bras for a bit of enhancement. I splashed out and bought a skin-tone bra as well. I only ever felt the need to wear an enhanced bra about twice after that surgery, but it was nice to know they were there, I suppose: a little like the earlier sleep-bra episode. I was very pleased indeed overall with the help I got and the purchases I made.

So now I had clothes, swimwear and underwear and I was ready to go on holiday as soon as I was allowed: and on the last trip to hospital to have the wound checked they said we could go. **YES!** It was a very rushed affair. We booked on Saturday to fly out the following Friday. My oncologist said, 'I did that once. You'll end up in Benidorm.' I think he knew that, after what we had been through, we might want to avoid 'club land'…

It was true that availability was scarce, but I had prayed that we'd find the right place because even our holidays are part of God's plans for our lives. When we booked, I wasn't at all sure: the only thing coming up on the agent's computer system that wasn't 'young people's club country' was a Greek island, and they told me it would be awfully hot. I don't *do* heat (or cold for that matter) terribly well, but this seemed the only real possibility in a welter of 'also-rans' – and it was affordable – so we booked it anyway.

The following Monday, I bumped into a church friend in the post office and told her that we were going to Poros. She knew Poros well, she said, and had been there herself. She was sure I'd like it. Would I like some information? Of course! We had wandered out into the market, still talking, when another friend from the same church group happened by. I told her my news. 'Well isn't that funny?' she said. 'I just happen to have this traveller's guide to Greece in my bag. I bought it for someone else but she's already got one. It's yours.' Given these events, I was definitely beginning to feel that the Lord was reassuring me that we'd booked the right holiday...

We packed bags and had begun to get into holiday mode when we hit a problem – 'no room at the inn' – or at least, no parking space at all at the airport for the week that we would require...not a single bay left anywhere and they were sorry. So were we! We investigated all sorts of possible solutions that included public transport or taxis, but all were prohibitive for one reason or another, often to do with expense. Then a thoughtful person from Gatwick phoned us back to tell us about a hotel that had a special arrangement: we could have a room there the night before we flew, parking for the duration of our holiday and transport to and from the airport, all for little more than the original cost of airport parking. Before that call we had not known such facilities existed. We snapped it up!

And so we were sorted. The hotel at the airport was very comfortable, even though with a four a.m. check in we were not long in bed – And then the flight was delayed! Eventually, however, we were airborne and relaxed – and the in-flight movie even turned out to be one I'd been longing to see. From Athens airport the coach transfer went very smoothly and we found ourselves on the ferry for the trip to the island, assisted by a very helpful rep. from the travel company.

I'd been apprehensive about this ferry transfer – I'd had a very dodgy one once in the Dominican Republic, but that's another story – but it was idyllic! The water was beautiful, with the sun playing on it, and we relaxed with shade and a drink watching islands apparently drift by. It was the perfect start to the holiday.

The seat beside me on the boat was vacant, and a lady of about my own age came and sat down. I discovered she was travelling alone, so I introduced her to Martin, sitting the other side of me, and we began to chat. I liked her immediately. She was warm, friendly and knowledgeable – she even knew Greek! Gradually, her story unfolded. She was going to Poros for her son, the younger of the two boys she had raised alone after the break-up of her marriage. He was half Greek and had dual English and Greek nationality and he had, very bravely, enlisted in the Greek Navy to do his national service, despite having only a smattering of the language. His passing out parade would take place this week, marking the end of his training, and my new friend, his mother, wanted to be there for him. From the first I was impressed by what I knew of both mother and son. I was delighted to discover that this lady was lodging in the same apartments as us, so we would be close neighbours for our stay.

Once installed, we had a terrific time. There was a super swimming pool very close by, and it was easy to walk into the local town, Askeli, or Poros Town itself. Yes, it was very hot, and once (and only once) I made the mistake of taking a longish walk in the middle of the day – my hands swelled up alarmingly and my fingers turned into bananas! I had to sit on the ceramic tiled floor with the electric fan we had hired full on me for about half an hour to reverse the process. But we learned to 'live Greek' and take a siesta – while I slept, Martin drew. He's actually a very talented artist, but he seldom has time to devote to sketching. He produced a closely detailed picture of the view from our apartment. These days, that sketch hangs in the study.

Every day we saw our new friend at least once. Sometimes we chatted at the pool, sometimes walked to town together. We found we got on really well and by mid-week we took an evening meal together in our apartment. Finding such a good friend to socialise with really enhanced our holiday. She took us to church; she was able to speak to the locals and find out when and where for us. Sunday mass was a beautiful experience, very close to the Orthodox tradition, though not entirely traditional, with many litanies and also much more that I recognised from my Roman Catholic background. There was a special reverence about it and we entered fully into the experience as the celebrants processed with the jewelled Bible, honouring the word of God. I felt entirely at home and wanted to receive communion but I didn't know how. I knew that these people believed in the real presence of Jesus in the bread and wine, as I did, and I felt deep inside that it would be right for me to receive communion here. If I did not do so, I would feel a sense of loss – but I was not sure what to do.

My new friend came to the rescue. Though she came from a different Christian tradition and did not wish to receive communion herself, she led me to the front of the church and made sure that I saw how to receive in the proper local manner. I will remember the sense of holiness that I felt throughout that service for the rest of my life. Sometimes, people like me who practise our faith regularly can lose that all-important sense of awe – of the holiness of God – through familiarity but here I felt it keenly, profoundly, and though I didn't speak the language, I did not need to: just to be immersed in the presence of God was a wonderful thing. The mass lasted about two hours, but both Martin and I were glad to have been there and neither of us begrudged the time at all. How could we? We hadn't really noticed it passing.

One day, Martin and I decided to visit Monastery. Most tourists on Poros go there at some point during their stay. The place is the site of an actual monastery, does have monks and a church, and is on the coast near to a beautiful bay. We visited the buildings, not the bay, climbing the stairs from the car park and passing through the doorway in the outer wall.

Correct mode of dress was essential: no naked arms or legs! There is a rail of wrap-around drapes at the entrance for those whose dress is inappropriate. Martin put on a long wrap-around skirt over his shorts, and I draped another over my shoulders, and we went in. We passed from the entrance porch into a courtyard and looked around us.

I had been told that there was a holy spring at this place, the waters of which are credited with healing people, through the power of God. I was anxious to find it and to take the water if possible. We did see some kind of faucet and a couple of tombs, but we did not really know what we were looking for or indeed at. I found a gate, held shut by a chain loop thrown over the post, and I opened it and walked through, into the back courtyard to the rear of the church. A few other tourists present at the time followed me. Having looked around, I came out of there, leaving the others behind me... And a young man called down from a first floor balcony in the adjoining living area, to say that visitors were not entitled to be in that area! I felt that I had to come clean and admit that I, now once more on permitted soil, had in fact led them all in! And this turned out to be another of those many experiences in life that God turns to our benefit, because the young man came down to talk to us.

He was a student of Theology, staying and studying at the monastery. He was American, not Greek, and had not lived a Christian life until coming to Greece a few years before and finding God. This remarkable person explained the iconography in the church to us. Suddenly I understood so much more. He was not angry about the incursion onto forbidden ground. He said he had to keep visitors out of those parts because the housekeeper was prone to become upset and agitated if they were in the wrong place. Having explained the icons, he led us to a special one we had not known about, credited with healing by the power of God. Many people had left offerings there; many of these were representations of the body parts for which they prayed for healing. I had no such offering that I could leave, having come unprepared, so I left an English coin and a guitar plectrum, hoping that would be a suitable representation of me... The young man told me they would be removed upon cleaning but I said that didn't matter – I know I left them there, and so does God!

One of the things that our new companion spoke to us about was the difference between Greek Orthodox tradition and Roman Catholicism. He explained that, though both churches can trace their tradition back to the disciples, and though both believe in the real presence of the Lord in the Eucharist, there is not inter-communion between the churches because of ancient and unhealed wounds. So sad that our humanity perpetuates the wounding of the Body of Christ! I was concerned and asked him, had I then, done a terrible thing in receiving communion on Sunday, when it had felt so right? The man's eyes positively danced with sparkles as he replied, 'Well I won't tell if you don't!' God's children know one another despite all the sorts of barriers our humanity throws up between us.

The healing spring turned out to be at the bottom of the monastery hill, near to the car park. I borrowed a glass from the small refreshment cafe and drank water from the spring. Martin did too. I later saw the young man filling a great water carrier for the monks; they drink the spring water all the time, apparently. The whole experience of the visit to this place had been special. In the quiet of the church we had prayed for some intentions very near to our hearts, as well as asking God for His continued healing and help for me. We had venerated God at the icon, drunk from the spring and felt ourselves to have been truly nourished by the Wellspring of Life Himself. Even when

I had been steering tourists in the wrong direction, God had been steering **me** in His way.

And now to something completely different! Martin had shown a real interest in the forthcoming passing out parade of the son of our new friend. Clearly he felt that such an event would be something rather special to behold. Walking past the naval base, it was often possible to glimpse things going on inside through the railings. He wondered if it would be possible to see something of the ceremonies in this way, or to ask our friend if it could ever be acceptable for mere members of the public to observe. I told him that I felt it would be unfair to ask her. This might be precious family time for her; a special time shared by herself and her son. I felt we must be careful not to intrude… Then she came looking for us and said, 'I've told the captain on the base all about you two and he said that you would be welcome to attend the ceremonies with me on Thursday if you would like to.' We were absolutely thrilled.

Suitably attired, semi-formally dressed but not over-the-top, and hopefully sufficiently lightly clad to cope with the searing mid-day heat, we went together to the base, equipped with cameras. There was a huge crush, made up of the family members of each young man on the base, jammed across the gates. People were conversing with varying degrees of excitement in Greek and many were seeking any available shade in the near vicinity as the sun rose ever higher. Shop doorways or the shadows of walls spilled over with people seeking their sanctuary. People craned to catch glimpses of what might be taking place on the other side of the railings. Martin and I felt privileged; we had no birthright to this event as all the others had.

An officer came and opened the iron gates, leading us through to a shelter giving standing room in the shade on the back parade ground. The many young men, smartly attired in white uniforms, were in serried ranks; dignitaries arrived with ceremony by helicopter. Four orthodox priests, clad from head to foot in their customary black, led prayers and the young men swore their oaths of allegiance. Speeches were made and demonstrations of the young men's new-found skills followed, with weapons drill and synchronised oarsman-ship. Despite the gruelling heat, it was all so very interesting, and we appeared to be the only non-Greek people there. Lacking means of communication, smiles and body language had often to suffice, but I wouldn't have missed it! Martin took photographs throughout, so that our friend and we ourselves would have a proper record of events. It was difficult to pick out her son among so many, but he made a valiant effort.

Suddenly it was all over. Dignitaries departed. The young men left to gather their kit, deposited earlier in bags on the front parade ground. Family members waited to accompany them off on leave. We waited for our friend's son to join us, which he did, and we returned to our holiday apartment building with one extra in tow. The holiday rep. was very accommodating; our 'extra' would be able come back to Athens with the tour party the following day at no additional cost, so all was sorted, and Martin was able to offer the lad a well-earned beer as we celebrated the completion of this part of his training.

That night we all ate out together at a local taverna, continuing our celebrations. The whole occasion had very much a family feel about it and being involved in these unexpected events had in many ways made our holiday – yet, after we returned home and wrote to our friend, she replied telling us how very much it had meant to **her** to have **us** around… Isn't it great that God can bring together members of the Christian family whenever and wherever there is need, regardless of differences of miles and culture? He had increased our joy and hers in this shared week and I have no doubt that it was His hand that brought us together.

Leaving the baking-bright beauty of Greece behind, we returned home, and within days I returned to work in earnest. No team teaching, now; just me and my classes, and the experience was one of mixed emotions. Some of my pupils were visibly relieved that we were back on track as they saw it, and made this clear to me. I properly reclaimed my classroom, my teaching base, and re-equipped it where necessary, helped partly by my father (who can supply almost anything, given adequate time, and legally too!) and partly by a sympathetic colleague who works wonders where computers are concerned and was ever patient with my then faltering expertise. I struggled – I still struggle – to keep things in proportion, aiming to remain on the premises until the day's marking and preparation were complete, so that I only took small amounts of work home, and I fought – I still fight – for a tidy classroom and the restoration and expectation of high standards in my territory, because I function best when I feel comfortable with the order around me. This is not a criticism of anybody else; some of my colleagues do an excellent job in what seems to me to be a sort of happy jumble, their skills often far surpassing mine – and they can always lay hands on what they want to find, however chaotic some of their systems appear to my eyes. For me, however, if the space is not tidy, neither is my mind, and I cannot cope.

Returning properly and hopefully finally, to work was a strange experience; mixed as I have said. All of my colleagues had been, without exception, totally, sympathetically, supportive, understanding and often loving. I was blessed in those with whom I worked. Even so, and through no fault of any of those people, the transition was in some ways difficult. I held a minor position of responsibility, and of course, during my absence others had covered for me. Upon my return, people were anxious not to over-face me, which was kind, but I could not be sure when I had totally taken up my reins once more, and I felt a certain guilt that some who did not receive the pay that I did were still perhaps shouldering part of my load on a lower income. And people who used to consult me about certain things had now adopted the very understandable habit of consulting others. This was entirely logical and I know there was no reason why I should have felt a certain degree of hurt, but that was the case, to my detriment. During my absence, job definitions had been redefined but mine was still very out of date for a very long time, since no one wished to put pressure on me…

So there it is. I was back in the same mould, doing what I have always done, in the place where, for almost nine years, I had always done it, BUT I WAS NOT THE SAME!

My body was different. I now looked very long and lean, whereas throughout my life before the diagnosis of cancer, I was very curvaceous – more so, it is true, than I ever wished to be. Maybe I even preferred my current shape, once dressed…

I had to learn to dress all over again, and had still not completely got to grips with my wardrobe. For the most part, my students seemed to have completely accepted the new me – many, I am sure, without really noticing a difference, though I did think that I noticed perhaps a small increase in those who (accidentally?) said 'Yes, Sir' in response to the register… Many of my friends and colleagues remarked that they genuinely felt I looked better without my old, ageing bust line. Certainly in many ways no bust is very much easier to dress and to live with than a huge bust was… And I turned down my prosthetic appointment. In theory now, I could have any size of bust I wanted. In practice I wanted to get out of bed and dress. I was through with self-assembly in the mornings. I know that it suits many women very well, and that is a terrifically important point, because each woman must be free to do what suits *her* best and makes *her* feel good and that *must* be facilitated, but for me, that means 'get up and go'. Despite making conscientious use of my referral to the gym, the two sides of my chest remained rather mismatched and I had to dress carefully. I thought I may later seek corrective surgery…

My hair was different. Always, for a very long time, hanging in long, straight, shaggy layers, then totally absent during chemotherapy, it was now in very short *wavy* layers. Even if I again grew it long, I didn't think it would ever be the same as before. I used to feel that flowing locks were mandatory for the identity of female guitarists, but I no longer had them, and many of my friends said that they preferred my hair short, and even that I looked younger… I did not know then what I planned to do long-term about my hair, and in any case, the helpful lady who had fitted my wig did say, 'We always tell ladies not to throw them away when they've finished with them, just in case…' I bought an afro-comb, suspecting it would give the best results on my new hair, and it proved to be the case.

Since treatment, my body functioned differently. Catapulted through the menopause, which, for me, was probably just beginning when my initial diagnosis of cancer was made, I now experienced regular hot flushes, though to a lesser extent, I am sure, than I would have if I had not been following the diet recommended by Professor Jane Plant. These episodes could make me feel suddenly very nauseous, weak and tired and they could be very embarrassing because I often needed to mop perspiration from my face. Hormone replacement therapy is not an option for someone with my medical history, so I just coped and relied on Grace.

Intimacy was different. I have been one half of the same loving relationship for all of my adult life. I was sixteen when I met my husband. My faithful Martin sustained me with his love throughout this experience and what we still share has grown through that, but my body chemistry was now very much altered, perhaps diminishing desire, and we had to learn to work at our relationship all over again (a duty not without its pleasures!) discovering new ways to express our love physically, not least because I lost my breasts! Things *were* different as a result, but no less meaningful and no less satisfying. How could they be, when our married love is grounded in and blessed by the love of God?

My mind worked differently. I do not know if it was because of the chemotherapy, the steroids I was given then, the Tamoxifen, or what, but my powers of thought changed. Sometimes I could not place a person I met. Sometimes, I moved to begin a task and then could not remember what I was about. Taking the minutes in meetings, I occasionally had to be prompted, as my short term memory failed me. Thankfully, my teaching seemed unaffected as my long-term memory seemed sound. I thought I might be a victim of BSE until I talked to a friend who has also had breast cancer and she described exactly the same experiences…

My faith had new dimensions. I always believed; I had received a life-changing conversion experience while still at school which enlivened the faith I had known since the cradle but, like many others I suspect, I previously often behaved as if I would live this life for ever. Now I could not know what the future held. (Of course, I never really did; such confidence was an illusion.)

Maybe my cancer was beaten. Maybe I should have total faith in this. God had told me many times: 'I know the plans I have for you... Plans to prosper you and not to harm you. Plans to give you hope and a future.' (Jeremiah 29, verse 11) I believed this. However, every time I got sick, I wondered if the cancer was returning... And if at some point it should, the same Lord who has always loved and cared for me will still love and care for me then. Those words give pause for thought; I can remember my mother speaking almost identical phrases as she bravely faced her own disease.

I do not think acknowledging the possibility of the return of the disease shows a lack of faith; rather, it is a testament to my humanity. I believe it is a natural consequence of what I have been through, and of having had such an aggressive strain of a potentially fatal disease, to be apprehensive about its possible return, even though I constantly acknowledge wholeheartedly the many and varied blessings showered upon me through this experience. God Himself knows only too well my human weakness. He made me, after all! Maybe it will be years before I can cease to be apprehensive in this way, so the important lesson is to live from day to day, in increased faith and trust. I haven't made it even now, but I'm gradually getting there, and the shining faith of some people I have encountered along the way whose disease has progressed, and who are still very sick, puts me to shame whilst helping to sustain me. I think back to that grapefruit, aim to live in trust, and ask that there be 'no maggots'!

I have so very much to be thankful for. God walked with me every step of the way through this experience and gave me strength in time of need as promised. He showed me sources of medical and dietary information which have been very helpful, in due season. He gifted me with an immediate family which enfolded me like a cocoon through the worst of it all and an extended family of aunts, uncles, cousins, nephews, nieces, in-laws, all of whom played their vital and loving parts. I did nothing to deserve any of this, and I am humbled by the amount of sheer goodness shown towards me.

Friends were often the raft upon which I rode these stormy waters – friends and clergy from the churches and prayer groups I attended, friends and colleagues from work, neighbours, or distant, long-standing friends who kept in touch; all kept my raft afloat… Special thanks were due to the friends with whom I still share the love of the music ministry: they will never know how much they gave me, or how much it meant.

In counting blessings, it is important not to forget the medical teams at the hospitals where I received treatment. From the greatest consultants and surgeons, through nursing staff and radiographers, to the kind ladies who cleaned the wards, they were constant in their conscientious caring, and the ever-patient breast care nurses deserve my special thanks.

What does the long-term future hold? I don't know. But then, I never did, though I may have thought so! Life is an adventure lived in episodes so much more eventful than the daily dose of 'soap' we so often take on board. I would be lying if I said that I did not have burdens of sorrow because of what happened. Sometimes I think I could cry for a week, even though to those around me the whole episode is now a thing of the past.

There is always great sorrow still to be worked through, perhaps because the emotions could not always be dealt with at the same time as the facts. I knew 'up' days and 'down' days and sometimes was easily moved to tears. But I live a life that is so much richer now. I have seen so many things I would never have seen, met so many people it has been my privilege to meet, received so much selflessly given and undeserved love… I know our God is a generous giver, pouring His wonderful gifts until the cup runs over – and then some! Somehow, this episode of sickness was right for me. God permits only that which will work for my greater good and the good of those around me, and I was slowly learning…am still learning…always learning… to 'let go and let God'. One day, I'll get there…but it is the tapestry of the journey that is the excitement and the work of the present…

Part Two

Learning Curves

and

Lollipops

To all intents and purposes, my confrontation with a rather nasty cancer was over. By the grace of God, I was well once more. I had undergone successful surgery to remove the tumour, then the breast, then, as a precaution, the other breast. I had undergone chemotherapy and radiotherapy. My hair, which had grown back curly after I lost it to the chemo, was once more straight and glossy. I was on a daily dose of Tamoxifen. Medical science had done all that it was able to do for me, helping me to fight an aggressive cancer that had begun to spread before it was diagnosed. God had done a great deal more.

Throughout the time when I was being treated, I had felt that I was receiving 'lollipops' from the Lord – sweet surprises that just appeared, some amazing, and some poignant – and some a great privilege. I wrote these events into my account of those days, for they made it all bearable and even worthwhile. With God, nothing is wasted.

Now I had resumed my life. I had changed my diet completely, in line with the recommendations of Professor Jane Plant, in her book 'Your Life In Your Hands'. A contact had recommended this book to me at a prayer meeting where our band were scheduled to play as music ministry. This, I am sure, was no accident. Now I was dairy free and full of soya and organic vegetables and fruits, and I felt well. I had longed for the return of that sense of well being, and I was really grateful to be back in the swing of things, doing all that I had been accustomed to do before and maybe more.

I had even changed my job. Previously a teacher in a good secondary school, I had often – so often – longed for the time to do more for those of my students who carried heavy burdens and struggled to cope. I knew this was a desire shared also by almost all of my colleagues and that the head was trying very hard to set appropriate counselling in place, along with alternative modes of education, but such things often progress slowly. Then I was offered a wonderful opportunity.

A teaching post became available within a supporting service which works alongside mainstream education, and after a successful interview, I was given a job within the service, in a centre a little like a mini school, but with the very great luxury of time so that I and others could give appropriate support to those who, for whatever reason, could not cope or were unable to remain in that mainstream education, since we taught only small groups or individuals.

I was very torn, because the school I had worked in meant a great deal to me. My colleagues had always been so supportive throughout my illness, my tutor group was a mixed bunch of super students of whom I was very fond (without exception!) and they had been so pleased to see me when I had returned to the classroom after my treatment. Now, only one school year down the line, I was moving on...

I know, though, despite the war of emotions, that the move was right. No experience in our lives is wasted, and my recent experiences had certainly changed me, physically, mentally and spiritually. It would have been wrong not to respond to those changes – not to move on.

There I was, then, the cancer behind, and a new life and a new job in front, with everything to live for. I discovered that, for me, there was still an issue that I needed to address...

After my first mastectomy, I had been very distressed by the way that I looked. I had always had huge breasts – 'G' or 'H' cup – and one such breast remaining was very hard to deal with, particularly as, due to my abnormally large breast size, achieving a good and comfortable result with prosthetics was not easy. Beside this, I had been told that, just like my original tumour, further cancer might be difficult to detect in a breast of this size, so I had, almost eagerly, consented to a second mastectomy.

After the second, precautionary mastectomy, I expected that my problems would be solved and the two sides of my chest would match each other, but the first mastectomy had been a radical one, removing also most of the pectoral muscle, and the second was much more conservative, leaving pectoral muscle and body fat. Though I looked fine when dressed in carefully selected crop tops, and though I chose to live as a flat-chested woman for two years and was adamant that I wanted no prostheses, (many women are very happy with these but I had hated 'assembling' myself on those mornings of treatment when I needed false breast and wig) I found it ever more difficult to live with what I now mentally referred to as my 'bomb site'.

It truly wasn't that I wanted breasts, particularly, but I desperately craved a better symmetry. One side of my chest was concave, literally to the ribs, and around this depression were a number of lumps of 'suspended' tissues, lumps of flesh that had once been part of something no longer there. The other side of my chest was more convex, with a very different scar, and an area of fullness along the bra line, created by loose skin. I asked advice in the breast clinic as to what I should do. As a result, I wrote to the chief consultant surgeon at the hospital where I had undergone my surgery.

Though I put my case in writing as eloquently as I could to that consultant, and though I ran the letter by the breast care nurses first and we agreed that it stated the case well, the consultant's written response seemed actually rather dismissive, even disputing some things which I knew to be correct about the present state of my chest: that left pectoral muscle tissue was missing, for example.

On the breast care nurse's advice, I made an appointment with him, so that he could see these things for himself. Clearly, he thought that the answer for people like me was to be found in external prosthetics.

These are a successful way forward for many people; such things are a matter of individual choice. Personally, however, I did not feel that this was an option I could live with. I do not think he was able to understand my position or to identify with my feelings over my body image. After a frustratingly brief discussion where all of this became clear, he asked me what I wanted and I, on the advice of the breast care nurses, asked for a referral to a plastic surgeon. At the time, there was one on the team at this, my local hospital. Unfortunately, he resigned, within the next few weeks, from the NHS. In his absence I was eventually referred to a hospital at some distance with a very good plastic surgery unit.

I went for a first consultation with the surgeon at this hospital, which was in a town twenty miles from my home, about two years after the second mastectomy. I asked this consultant, a gentle man who immediately inspired confidence, to do anything he could to neaten up my chest, and explained that, above all, I desired a greater degree of symmetry, and that I did not intend to wear external prostheses.

He examined me very thoroughly, sitting and standing, examined my tummy, clearly assessing how much donor tissue there might be there, and had me perform an abdominal 'crunch' while he was so doing, presumably to feel what was working muscle and what was fat, then he asked me to dress and move from the examination room to a smaller office for consultation.

Once there, he put a startling proposition to me. He said, in as many words, 'You're going to go through it anyway, whatever we do, so we won't mess about. This is what I propose...'

What he outlined was quite something – a procedure called D.I.E.P. flap breast reconstruction. The initials stand for Deep Inferior Epigastric Perforator. Leave you reeling? It did me, too, but essentially the operation was described to me as follows: Skin and its underlying fat would be harvested from my abdomen, with a supporting blood supply dissected out from the underlying muscles. The muscles themselves would not be taken, so I would not be at risk of a hernia. The donor skin would then be fashioned into two eye-shaped pieces, and attached to the two sides of my chest to create new breasts. This would mean attaching the veins taken with the donor skin to veins in my chest area, thus establishing a new blood supply to support each flap (area of donor skin). Veins would have to be stitched very delicately to others if this was to be successful.

This microsurgery requires infinite care and patience. It is wonderful, in that it does not require the use of any kind of implant. From the outset, having had angry skin reactions to silicon when worn as an external prosthesis, I was adamant that I wanted none inside me! This had been one of my key starting points: my own body tissues or nothing! I was blessed, in that I had been referred to a team that would undertake such a complex 'own body tissue' reconstruction. I knew the team was trustworthy because my oncologist had told me that he wouldn't allow me to go to anyone that he didn't trust, and he would vet anyone the surgical team referred me to, and satisfy himself that they could be trusted!

Even so, I felt that this sounded like a huge undertaking. I had told my new employers that I might, at some point, need minor surgery for a tidy up. I had not envisaged anything like this, and nor, I was sure, had they. This sounded like very major surgery. The consultant explained that it involved vast areas, yes, but in a superficial way: they'd not be going near major organs, as the whole procedure was just skin and fat deep. I would be likely to spend six and a half hours under anaesthetic, seven to ten days in hospital, and I would need six weeks off work. He very wisely told me that I was to make no decision at that time, but must go away and think about it, discussing everything with my husband who had been present throughout the consultation, and return to see him again in one month's time.

Before leaving I raised what I felt to be an important question. 'What you propose is without doubt a big undertaking. It is about three years since I had cancer. I may only have about two more years to live, or I may live to be ninety. Is it wise to embark on this road now?' His reply was very direct: 'My money would be on ninety, and in any case, if you had limited time left, then I think you should have this procedure sooner rather than later.' I believe there is in fact good statistical evidence that women who have reconstructive surgery often do better long term than those who do not. Maybe that was what lay behind the consultant's response.

I left for the car park with my head still reeling. It sounded exciting but huge. What about the risks…the family? What about the time off work? I was in turmoil. I put my hand on the handle of the passenger side door of the car, intending to open it and at that precise moment remembered something I had long ago 'put on the back burner'.

Many months before, when I was on chemo, I had been prayed over by a priest with a healing ministry, a visitor from abroad. He had, at that time, asked our music ministry to play for an event to take place in the coming weekend. We had expressed doubts about whether we would be able to make it, due to my sickness and commitments the others had, but he had said, 'You will be there.' In the event this had proven totally impossible as I had cut my finger very badly, had to have a course of antibiotics, and could not possibly play guitar! Therefore I had decided that, in this instance, he had clearly been mistaken and I thus discounted something else that he had said to me at the same time; words which now came very clearly back into my head as I stood with my hand to the door of the car: 'God is going to give you a new breast. I see a substance like milk running through your breast.'

I had always known that God could, and would if he chose so to do, make me whole again. In an instant, just like that! Once, I had even looked to see if He'd done it. Now I began to wonder if this was it. Was this the way He would restore me?

Knowing that we had a lot of thinking to do, Martin and I began to talk in the car as we journeyed home. What the consultant had said had sounded good and promising – but major – and there was no getting away from the fact that it was essentially a cosmetic procedure, since I was now well. But I could not imagine that anyone would deny a person who had, say, a facial disfigurement – perhaps a divided lip or a burn scar – the right to have corrective surgery, given the chance. My disfigurement was just as great or greater, even though usually concealed under carefully selected clothing. My husband and I both had to look at it every day. Given the chance, it felt right to correct it. Could it be that the outcome of this amazing microsurgery, fastening veins to veins and creating a new pattern of blood flow, would lead to the fulfilment of the visiting priest's prophecy: 'a substance *like* milk, flowing through your breast'?

One thing that caused me concern a little later was the feeling that we had largely made the decision based on our gut reactions before I felt we really turned it over to prayer. I wished that my first recourse had been to seek God's will in this and felt that perhaps it had not. Realising that, despite the month we had been given, we seemed to have decided in favour of surgery fairly quickly, I began to pray about it somewhat retrospectively and to search for wisdom.

I think that, for those who try to walk with God, a gut feeling that something is right is probably a reliable indication. After all, if you try to live your life under His guidance, God is not going to play tricks upon you, trip you up, or hold out hope and snatch it away…but I put the question of surgery into my daily prayer, and I sought confirmation through talking to my family and Christian friends and gauging their reactions, feeling that God would also give them wisdom, and through them show me His will. Almost to a man, they were positive, feeling that it was not God's will for me to live with that degree of disfigurement.

One person told me the story of a priest who had had a similar dilemma, due to a very disfiguring abdominal scar, and had felt in prayer that God wanted him to take the opportunity to have it fixed. My father spoke of the sorrow that my mother's and my stepmother's mastectomy scars had recalled to mind, and the joy he would have felt to have seen them restored. A few spoke of how they would never have the courage to undergo surgery that was not essential to their health, but they did not suggest that *I* should not undertake it; they merely seemed to think that I was brave to consider doing so. This, by the way, I refute. If something is right, then it is God who gives us the necessary courage at the right time.

One month after the first appointment, I told the surgeon I would like to go ahead. He immediately suggested January – about a month away, and I was again worried about the implications for my job. It was not possible to schedule for the school holidays, the consultant said, because operating lists were subject to change in response to emergencies, and this made the whole exercise of planning in this way futile. I asked for the grace to check things with my place of work. Here I found only understanding and encouragement, but I was begged to make it any time *after* January, since there was an inspection due that month and, as the surgery was non-urgent, I was happy to comply. I told the surgeon's secretary any time from February onward.

I began to address another issue that concerned me. I had been told I may need blood transfusion during the operation and I found I was worried about this. I have no ethical objections of any kind; in fact I used to be a blood donor, but I guess I was just anxious, probably irrationally, about receiving blood. Relatively recently, at that time, there had been items in the press about transmission of variant CJD and about HIV contaminated blood... I researched the possibility of laying down my own blood in advance, so that I could be transfused with it, should it be necessary. This is perfectly possible. It is called autologous transfusion and is quite routinely done, where people apply and fill in the appropriate paperwork. Once the application is received, each case is assessed on its merits and in that way the suitability of the individual for this process is assessed.

At the same time that I was applying, a very good friend who was facing surgery for prostate cancer also applied, since this seemed a good idea to him when I talked about it. In an ironic turn of events, he was accepted and began to lay down his blood, and I was rejected as unsuitable! Why? Because, I was told, my veins (notoriously difficult to access, it is true) were not suitable and the level of iron in my blood was too low! Well, that told *me*! The surgeon said that he felt my fears relating to donated blood were irrational – it wouldn't bother *him* to receive it – and Martin and I concluded that the possibility that I may have to receive donated blood was not a reason not to go ahead. Though the fear that surrounded this for me remained real, I began to pray for anyone giving blood that I may be about to receive.

I was given a surgery date in March and my life became frantic. Though I had only been in post since September, I was committed to my job and to the students. I had been warned I would need six weeks to recover, so that meant developing a system to devise and leave six weeks' worth of suitable work in some kind of foolproof and accessible format for every child that I taught. At that time I was teaching six subjects at secondary level and every student was on an individual education plan! I threw myself into the extra work, often remaining in my classroom long after hours, which was truly exhausting at times. As the date approached, I prepared the students, showing them where they would be able to find everything they and their cover teachers would need. I also found, as far as I was able, staff that would be willing to cover for me, and briefed the cover teachers.

Then the bomb was dropped.

It was Thursday. I was due to enter hospital on the following Monday. While I was teaching in the afternoon, the phone rang. The call was from the surgeon's secretary, who was very sorry to have to tell me that she was ringing to cancel my operation, due to the emergency admission of a woman with active cancer who could not wait. This person's right to priority was utterly undeniable, but I was so gutted that I had to cut the phone call short, explaining that I knew it was no one's fault, but in the circumstances I found it hard to remain calm and polite, having been psyched up for Monday, and having done *so* much exhausting preparation at work! I felt churlish that I was unable to respond any better, but I knew that this kindly lady understood.

A colleague took me out of the school building for a walk on the common. I was distraught. I had been told there would now be a long delay, because the surgeon was due to go abroad for a few weeks and his list was full up to his departure date and for a short period after his return. In other words, all that work I had prepared, I would now have to teach, being the next part of each curriculum, and the preparation process would have to begin all over again! The method I had devised was set up. I would live that method myself for the time being, then re-stock the folders for the stretch when, finally, I *would* be gone…

The colleague I walked with that day gave me the strength and perspective I needed as we talked. We agreed that things like this happen for a reason. We agreed that God must be in this somewhere. I knew this, I really did, but at this particular time it gave me little comfort. So many friends and family had been in touch to offer their support also, and they all needed to be informed it was now off. It was such a depressing task, as was the thought of revising those folders!

I think the majority of people were really surprised when I told them what had happened, but I benefited from a terrific emotional blanket, both in fact and in prayer. I was particularly touched that our priest suggested a date when he would give me the sacrament of the sick in preparation for the operation. I received the anointing late one evening in the side chapel of the church, surrounded by a few close friends who were praying for me. I felt even more reassured that God was with me and would sustain me.

The time that I now had to wait gave me other opportunities. I was able to teach my G.C.S.E. candidates right up until study leave began. I did not have to feel that I was running out on them. (This would not, of course, have been the case. Cover of an extremely high calibre had been arranged, but I did feel a sense of responsibility, and this was a responsibility I was now able to fulfil. In this way, God's timing was instantly proven far superior to mine.) The other thing I was able to do was something the surgeon, a leading man in his field in every sense, had suggested long before; I was able to find time to look up the procedure on the Internet.

When I did this, I was truly surprised at what I found. I was not looking at promotional sites, but medical ones and some giving patients' own accounts regarding what they had undergone. I found everything to be very encouraging indeed. The medical sites clearly detailed the operation I was to have, with photographs in colour of each stage of the surgery. The patients' write-ups were very positive, and their photographs after surgery looked great. I tried to get information on some problems the surgeon had told me about, principally flap failure, (this is the death of the tissue which has been relocated during the operation, usually due to a problem in blood supply) but could find nothing negative. It was a shock to find that I was

actually saying aloud to myself, 'Oh, I **want** this!' I had not, up
to this point, known the strength of my own feelings.

I was now more confident. The revised lesson planning at work
was going better than I had anticipated, because the structure
was in place; only the actual lessons needed revising, since the
timetables, records and notes remained largely the same. At one
of the weekly prayer meetings, a friend told me that she felt the
Lord had said, 'Behold, I make all things new,' – confirmation of
what I had felt He had been telling me for some time. Indeed, I
already had a working title of 'All Things New' for this second
part of my written account of my journey. The strong desire I
had experienced when I surfed the net for information on the
surgery had helped to confirm that this was indeed the right
path for me, and I was intensely grateful.

It is impossible to escape the fact that all surgery carries risk
and I couldn't help a degree of continuing anxiety. When I had
cancer, the risk of surgery was negligible, compared to the risk
of declining it, but this operation I was looking at was elective;
I didn't **have** to have it. And it did carry risks. The surgeon
had said that I could **die** (admittedly this was unlikely), that I
could suffer a thrombosis, that there was a possibility of flap
failure if the transplanted skin didn't 'take' and a possibility of
infection. And there remained the issue of blood transfusion.
In the light of all this, the decision to go ahead really was a
major one. It helped to look into the bedside mirror at night
and remember that if I didn't take this opportunity I'd look
like that or worse (time and gravity do no favours) for the
rest of my life, however long that was, and I'd always wonder
whether I should have taken the chance for change when it
was offered to me. Those who saw my naked chest were all

of the opinion that 'that needs sorting out'. So was I, I once again decided.

I received a second call from the consultant surgeon's secretary. How would I feel about being on video? This was not a question I had expected in this context, but the reason for it became clear as she explained. I had already been knocked back once, because urgent surgery always takes precedence over elective surgery. This could, in theory, happen once or perhaps twice more before hospital policy dictated that, on my next due date, I **had** to be admitted, no matter what. For me, since I had the obligation to set work for my students, any further delays would mean mountains of further preparatory work. However, the hospital had a teaching day coming up in May, when outpatients would be closed and the area filled with doctors who would be watching proceedings in several operating theatres on video. Selected teams would be working on selected operations in those theatres, and I could be one of the surgical cases for that day if I was willing. Would I think about it and call the secretary next day? The beauty of this would be that I could not, if selected, be cancelled. Martin and I decided that there was not much to think about, in fact. It seemed obvious that, with so many observers, I would get excellent care. Would my consultant be operating? Oh, yes, he'd be there. We accepted the May date.

My workmates were great. Cover teachers for my lessons were once again arranged. The head of our unit and the head of the service were each immensely positive. One person expressed interest in the fact that this was cosmetic surgery, but once I explained, she realised it was not to be like a breast enlargement job! As I have said, surgery for facial disfigurement such as a divided lip for example, is essentially elective, even cosmetic, but no one would suggest that a person with such a disfigurement should just live with it! I assured those who were curious that my chest was every bit as disfiguring! Granted, it was mostly hidden by clothing most of the time, but *I* had to see it every day, as did my husband, and that was why I felt it was right to take this chance to 'sort it out'.

Around two weeks (maybe a little longer) before the operation date, I had to go to the hospital for blood tests, preliminary examinations and to sign my consent. A doctor once more explained the form that the operation would take, answered my questions, filled out forms and showed me where to sign my consent. I also saw an anaesthetist, a lady, who described the surgery I was about to have as 'a beautiful operation' and explained to me that it would be unlike any previous surgery I had experienced (I invariably wake up shivering with cold) because this time, in order to keep my veins nice and full, they would be pouring warm liquids into them, and keeping my body warm also. Fluid *in* means fluid *out*, so I would need a catheter. It all began to feel like an even greater undertaking than I'd thought, but this anaesthetist was very reassuring. She had seen many successful similar surgeries (though perhaps none identical) and though there had been complications with some, they had always been sorted out. She was confident of a successful outcome for me.

I was also sent to the Medical Photography Department for 'before' photographs to be taken. This was a strange experience, as my chest was no thing of beauty and I felt raw and exposed in front of the male photographer, who was, for obvious reasons, keen to record accurately every unattractive detail. His manner was gentle and totally appropriate. He apologised for being male (as if he could help it?) and for the fact that his female colleague had stepped out. He asked whether it would be O.K. if he took the pictures or would I rather wait? There really was no reason to be difficult, and so I stood half naked before him with my husband as chaperone, and the pictures were taken. Why would anyone need a chaperone with a chest as unappealing as mine? It certainly had no power to attract!

Shortly before the surgery date, the consultant himself called me. He wished to make a small change. Though he would be present on the teaching day, he would not personally have been able to perform my operation, which he would like to do. Would I therefore please come to the hospital one day later? I was more than happy to comply. Obviously I was not now to be a star of theatre and screen for a day (at least from the neck down!), but I was certainly to be in the best hands.

The run-up to surgery had caused me one other concern. I was taking various supplements, which I believed to be helpful in maintaining my health and preventing a recurrence of breast cancer. Daily, I took red clover, selenium with vitamins A, C, and E, often Brewer's Yeast and I sprinkled golden linseeds on my cereal for the omega 3 fatty acids they contain. My surgeon had once had a harrowing experience when he treated a previous patient who had taken a range of supplements. The team had been unable to staunch bleeding during surgery because something in the supplements the lady had taken had seriously affected the clotting factors in her blood. Unable to establish exactly what had caused the problem, the team did not want any of their future patients to be taking any non-prescription supplements at the time of surgery or for three or four weeks beforehand. Thus I was asked to stop taking anything other than Tamoxifen before my first surgery date (which, of course, was cancelled) and had only just resumed my regime when I was asked to stop once more. I did feel a little anxious about this. I knew that the preparations I had to make at work and at home before surgery had put me under stress and I knew that I needed to be as well as possible before surgery. I wasn't sure that stopping my supplements was the best way, but I had to be guided by the consultant surgeon's advice.

Just before I was due to enter hospital, I asked Martin to take some honest, 'full-on' photographs at home, using the digital camera. 'I want something to look at when I feel lousy, to remind myself why I did this,' I told him. He took the photographs, with me standing naked to the waist, in our bedroom, and then, for the time being, I forgot about them.

Somewhat harassed, in a flurry of final preparations, I developed a cold. I was not entirely over it on the day of admission and I was terrified that I would be sent home. In the event, I was examined, found not to be too bad, and sent for a chest x-ray. If this proved clear, things would go ahead. My blood tests also had to be repeated, since they had been done two weeks before. This is always a harrowing proceeding, because, since the chemo, my veins are awful. In addition, since the lymphectomy under my left arm, only the right arm can be used anyway – but we got the blood out somehow. Once these preliminaries were over, I found myself at my allocated bed ('We **will** find you a pillow later, we promise!') and I set out, on the table and locker, cards and good wishes and a little floral garland, a gift from a colleague. I had received encouragement from family, workmates, fellow Christians and many kind friends. I remain **so** grateful, to this day, for all of that support. Sometimes cancer patients find friends can be less in evidence; they feel awkward and don't know what to say. Actually, you don't need to say anything: just **be** there!

And through the whole admission process my faithful Martin was at my side, unfailing in the strength he poured into me through his own calm confidence. I had asked him so many times if this was the right thing to do and he always responded that he believed it was. Now that I was in the hospital, it was time to 'let go and let God' and allow events to take their course.

My fellow patients were awaiting various plastics procedures. Many needed tendons reconnected after injuring hands, in order to regain function. Some needed bad breaks in bones to be set. Many more needed skin grafts over ulcers that would not heal. There were four of us in the bay where I spent that first night: two 'legs', one 'arm' and me. We were of widely varying ages, but the atmosphere was pleasantly sociable.

I discovered that I had received two identical prayer cards designed for people receiving in-patient treatment, one from the chaplaincy team at the hospital and one from a friend who, with me, was involved in Sunday radio services at our local hospital. (The hospital I was now in felt far from local; it was about an hour's drive from home.) Feeling unsure of the likely response, I offered one of these cards to one of the other patients with whom I had struck up a conversation. She was eager to accept it and obviously pleased to receive it. How easy it would have been for me just to keep the two, 'minding my own business' rather than risking a possible adverse reaction. More and more I feel there are few things that genuinely happen by accident… Now each of us, waiting for surgery, had a card which, amongst other things, carried a 'prayer before an operation' printed upon it. That had to be a good thing!

Sometime during that afternoon's proceedings, I had been given a leaflet, written by a leading member of the physiotherapy department, entitled 'D.I.E.P. Flap Reconstruction Of The Breast', and advised to read it through. It proved helpful, giving information about the surgery itself, what to expect upon waking from the anaesthetic, what my limitations would be and what exercises I should do, once given permission, to help myself to recover. I found that I referred to this leaflet many times whilst in hospital and frequently after returning home. Something tangible and easily accessible to the anxious reader is a real gift. I wish more hospitals would issue this type of information on a broader scale than seems to be the case.

Purposeful members of the surgical team came to see me that evening to mark up my tummy. They had a strange little device attached to a thing like a pen. When the 'pen' passed over the skin of my tummy above my blood vessels, it was possible to hear from the device the sound of my blood coursing through my veins. When a good vein was located, the sound was louder and the site of that vein was marked on my skin in black felt tip. Six or so such sites were located and marked, and some lines were also drawn onto my chest, apparently marking as closely as possible what had once been my natural breast line. Looking now like an ancient map marking sites to dig for buried treasure, I was to go to theatre early next morning.

To my surprise, that evening I learned two things. The first was that even my Tamoxifen had to be stopped until the surgeon told me that I could restart it. (Now I felt my entire 'anti-cancer umbrella' was gone! How weak we are, and how we place our faith in human measures! God was still God! I believed He had led me here. Where was my faith?)

The second thing was to be a problem throughout my stay in that hospital. I wished to keep to my dairy free diet. I had followed the advice in Professor Jane Plant's book 'Your Life In Your Hands' as closely as I was able ever since it had been recommended to me shortly after diagnosis. My oncologist had said, 'You will not do yourself any harm and you may do yourself good', adding that trials investigating the effects of such a regime upon the outcome in cancer patients were still underway and a conclusive report still awaited. He obviously felt there was merit in Professor Plant's research and conclusions and so did I.

The diet had never been a problem when hospitalised before, but apparently it might be now... That night, the canteen eventually provided a piece of chicken, a jacket potato and some peas, so I was fine. Later, I did not fare so well! In other hospitals there is a menu card system. Often the card has helpful information beside the choices, such as a 'heart friendly' symbol, or the words 'low fat' or 'vegetarian'. They frequently also have 'ethnic' choices, so that I have, in the past, selected a dish which is perhaps intended for people whose religion requires a vegan diet. In this hospital, for the midday and evening meals, a trolley of food was sent up. There were a number of appetising choices on the trolley and the menu was often imaginative; celery and red pepper soup, for example.

Unfortunately, it was seldom possible to work out what food upon that trolley would definitely be dairy-free. Had the fish been basted with butter? Had batter been made with milk or water? Were the vegetables garnished with butter? Was there milk or cream in the soup/sauce? The really difficult thing about all this was that, even when domestic staff contacted the kitchen to try to answer these questions, the staff down there could not answer, since ingredients were listed only on the huge outer carton used for delivery and they had made up whatever the substance was from a smaller, inner carton giving only the name of the product and no list of ingredients. Even when they tried to send 'safe' food separately, there were unanswered questions. If fish comes with carrots and mashed potatoes, is it possible to be sure that the carrots have not been glazed with butter, or that there is no butter, milk, or margarine containing milk solids, in the mash?

One day, the kitchen staff asked over the phone whether I ate fish (as in salmon/tuna) or eggs. I responded that I very happily ate both. Curiously, they then sent up a jacket potato with baked beans and a side salad! I ate this, and I enjoyed it, but I found the logistics behind such events difficult to grasp. In the end, we concluded that the kitchen in this hospital was not really geared to certain special diets (though I did see the occasional carton labelled 'gluten free' on the food trolley) and it was obvious that the daily feeding of so many patients was, in any case, a mammoth task, difficult enough without trying to sort me out!

There was even one day when someone down there, trying hard to please, sent stir-fried beef, which smelt wonderful. I was really tempted, but according to the advice in the book that I followed, the harmful biochemicals that are in milk (oestrogens, prolactin, IGF1) are often in the mass-reared beef as well. And, like many people, in these post BSE days, I was suspicious of non-organically raised beef. I could not bring myself to eat it…

All of my problems would have been solved had there been a vegan option on the daily menu, but there wasn't, and it just wasn't reasonable to expect the harassed kitchen staff to get to grips with my diet, so in the end we made our own arrangements, and Martin, bless him, actually managed to bring me a hot meal in a container each evening and a sandwich to put into the fridge for the following day's lunch. Breakfast was not a problem; I provided the soya milk and they provided the Weetabix! From time to time my friends, always very supportive of my efforts to take some personal responsibility in maintaining my health, cooked for me to save Martin a job, and it was one of these friends who supplied the 'stay-hot' container, too. Humbling to realise that people were prepared to go to such lengths for my benefit…

It probably seems strange, or precious, or picky, that I was apparently being so difficult about food, but please remember I had been told to stop taking all of the supplements that I believed helped to keep cancer at bay, including Tamoxifen. I had been on my dairy free diet now for almost three years. At home, I ate organic lamb and chicken, but not beef or pork, (except, rarely, bacon) due to the methods by which these are bred and raised. I loved vegan food and ate it often. This hospital was, after all, in a large cosmopolitan town. Many people who enter a hospital owe their ethnic origins to Africa or the Indian sub-continent and some of these people *are* vegan. I asked the nursing staff what such patients do about food, and was told that their family members bring it in, so there you have it! We did the same.

Early in the morning, on the day after my admission, I was taken to theatre. I had been told my operation would take about six and a half hours. In fact, it took much longer; twelve hours, and I cannot remember much of what happened immediately beforehand. I suspect this is at least in part due to the length of time I was under anaesthetic. I do recall that I was treated with reassuring kindness and that the anaesthetist had visited in advance and was very considerate also. Then came the 'Here we go, Lord,' moment that begins every operation – the time when I know that it's just me and the Everlasting Arms – and I lost consciousness…and a whole day!

I know that, after surgery, I went into the recovery room, but I can recall very little until I was once more on the ward. I was lying on my back, with a pillow under my knees. I was covered by, but not wearing, my fetching theatre gown, and I had the beautiful regulation white anti-thrombosis stockings on my legs. At some point, I was also given 'Flowtron' boots, which slowly inflate and deflate in order to assist the circulation in the legs while the patient is immobile. Underneath the gown laid across my body, there was a 'gamgee'. This is a thick piece of padding, rather like cotton wool, and it extended over the whole of my chest area, giving protection and warmth. I knew that I was catheterised, and I had a drip up and five drain tubes leaving my body: two from the abdomen, one from each side of my chest and one extra one, of a different type, from the side of the new left breast.

One thing I *do* remember is that very soon after I was returned to the ward the consultant came to the foot of my bed and explained that there was one area of my chest that he hadn't managed to sort out, but I was not to worry; they'd do it with a small implant later! Implant? What had I said about *that* before? I wasn't really able to take in what he was saying, but I knew even then that I didn't want that implant, or to contemplate further surgery at this point!

Nurses came at least every hour to 'check my flaps' – to make sure that the newly transplanted skin was remaining healthy and had sufficient blood supply. They were also very attentive to *all* my possible needs; sips of water, a wipe of my face, a mouthwash, a tissue. My bed was not in the bay it had previously occupied, but right beside the nurses' station, curtained all around to give me some privacy, and it was not long before it was moved again into a private room. I had morphine, through a PCA (Patient Controlled Analgesia system; you press a button and the pain goes away). I had an oxygen mask, soon replaced by a lighter tube under my nose for my comfort, and, under all of this, I drifted in and out of sleep for some while. I was unable to do anything else. That twelve-hour anaesthetic had really knocked me for six and even my speech was severely affected. It seemed I could only speak very slowly, and my voice was more of a whisper or croak than its usual strident self!

There were very strict instructions at this time as to how I was to lie, and what movements I might and might not make. My pillows had to be at a particular angle, almost flat at first and only gradually being raised over a number of days to let me sit up. There were more pillows under my knees to keep my legs bent, and a roll of bedding known as a 'donkey' at my feet to prevent me from straightening my legs. For weeks, in fact, I had to sleep as if in a chair, in this folded position. Initially, I also had to rest my arms on pillows positioned as supports.

One of the nurses, who attended to me while I was still bed-bound and catheterised, washed me well, and then, very kindly, agreed to wash my hair. This seemingly impossible feat was achieved by stripping the top end of the bed to the plastic-covered mattress and tilting the foot end of the bed up and the head end down. In this way, water could be poured into my hair and would then run off into a bowl at the top of the bed. Ingenious! And did I feel better for it!

At some stage during this time, I was visited by a physiotherapist. She asked me if I could take a deep breath. Not sure that I understood the way she was demonstrating, I asked if I could do it *my* way, and, though she seemed a little confused by the question, she said any way would be fine. I have had some voice training and breathing exercises were a very important part of this, so drawing upon that experience, I took my breath as I had been taught. Apparently, it impressed her, because another 'physio' later told me I had seemingly just 'breathed in and in'! After a major or a long operation, it is very important to ensure patients breathe deeply to oxygenate the blood and help to clear the anaesthetic gasses. My oxygen saturation was checked very frequently over the next few days and I was encouraged to continue the deep breathing. Very soon, the levels were deemed to be good enough for me to come off the supporting oxygen and I was given a little plastic contraption a bit like a peak-flow meter to encourage me to make the effort to continue aiming for greater chest inflation, particularly in the lower lobes of the lungs. This I used throughout my stay in hospital.

During the first days after the surgery, as I was drifting between sleep and wakefulness, a piece of music called 'The Father's Song' was with me, going round and round in my head, almost whenever I was awake and aware. This song tells of how God the Father rejoices over his children with singing, and of how He has called us and cares for us. It is based on a Bible verse from Zephaniah. To have it as a constant mental backdrop was very reassuring indeed and I don't believe it was a coincidence. Strength and encouragement come when we need them.

Sooner by far than I would have wished, I had no option but to think again about surgery, because there was a problem with, of all things, my navel! The skin and fat that was needed to rebuild my chest had been taken from my tummy. The incision was right across the front of my body from the side of the left hip to the side of the right, below the bikini line. The tissue taken was four or five inches in depth, so the rest of the skin on my front was stretched and joined, giving me a 'tummy tuck'. My navel had been preserved in its original position and a neat hole had been made for it, into which it had been beautifully stitched, but, due to poor blood supply, my 'tummy button' died! It turned vaguely black and looked very strange. It would have to be removed.

Two days, then, after my original twelve-hour surgery, I was once more in the operating theatre, this time fully conscious, while, under local anaesthetic, my navel was excised. I tried not to look, but you have to close your eyes or look somewhere! It would have seemed rude to close my eyes; the team members were chatting to me. I confess I saw some things I wish I hadn't, and the whole experience was not a pleasant one. Queasy anyway, this served to make me feel still worse. Apparently, the loss of the navel is a complication that sometimes happens, but I had not been warned of this possibility… I felt that, to the surgical team, compared to the wonder of what they had positively achieved for me with God's help, this little negative blip was 'small potatoes'. I, however, was distressed by it. That navel had been part of me for more than fifty years and I was sorry to see it go! The whole proceeding left me sad and downhearted, as well as sickened.

Back in my private room, I was again recovering. The catheter and my drains were each removed as soon as they were no longer needed. I was encouraged to move around a bit. I had time to contemplate what had been done to me. Lacking a full-length mirror, I had not seen my new breasts. I could see very little in the head-and-shoulders mirror above the hand basin. I could only gain some impression of my appearance from looking down at my body. I had, however, a sense that my two new 'boobs' were rather unequal! Remember that, prior to surgery, I had had a radical mastectomy to the left side, largely removing the pectoral muscle as well as all breast tissue and body fat. On the right side, I had had a much more conservative mastectomy, preserving the pectoral muscle and a quantity of body fat. Given all of this, an uneven result is hardly surprising. Anxious about my appearance, I frequently asked the same young nurse if I would be pleased with the result of my surgery. Would I feel it had been worth it? She was sure that I would.

One day, she was accompanied by a young male, a student nurse, when the question again came up. She offered to fetch a mirror and to sit with me while I had a good look. In order to spare my blushes, the young student was preparing to make himself scarce. I asked her to let him know that he would be welcome to sit with us. How else was he to learn, to gain insight, to develop empathy? So it was that three of us sat down to have a good, long, critical look.

Yes, the result was uneven, but there was no denying that I looked a lot better with breasts than without. Lots of women have uneven breasts, anyway. The nurse herself confided that she used padded bras and put both pieces of padding into one side of the bra in order to even her own bust line up. She felt that there was nothing here that the right bra wouldn't sort. For my part, I was relieved. Even at this stage, with raw scars, I looked better than I had expected. I was somewhat reassured.

By evenings, at this stage of events, I would generally be tired and very sore. Things were extremely busy on the ward one day. I buzzed for a nurse to help me to prepare for sleep because I was very uncomfortable and wished to retire early, but no one came for over two hours. (There were assistants on the ward who could answer calls but had to refer certain things to the nurses. The nurses were first busy, then 'in handover', which is why none came to me.)

I was wearing an abdominal binder to support the wound across my bikini line. It was a strong, elastic support and I was grateful for it. I had been told to wear it whenever I was out of bed, and had been encouraged to get up and walk around as much as possible, but **not** to attempt to stand up straight yet, or to raise my elbows above my head, or stretch to reach for anything. Any of these could damage areas of my body that had recently been sutured. Upon returning to bed for sleep, I was still under strict instructions as to how I might lie.

The nurse finally arrived to help me prepare for sleep and, in doing so, took off the binder. Underneath it, my discomfort was explained. I had an extensive and impressive red rash, from below my navel wound to the tops of my legs. Concerned, the nurse called the doctor.

When the registrar came, she was not sure whether the rash was due to allergy or infection. I was on Erythromycin as a preventative measure, to guard against the latter eventuality. She felt that, to be on the safe side, I should also take Flagyl, another powerful antibiotic. I felt that the rash looked allergic rather than infected, so I was given an antihistamine tablet, which would help if this was the case. I was already on iron tablets, and, with this strange cocktail making my queasy stomach rebel, I tried to sleep.

The following morning, I felt I had fearful flatulence, but the truth turned out to be far worse. Already feeling really ill, I now seemed to have lost all control of my bodily functions and therefore all dignity. In abject and embarrassed misery, and still in pain, I spent a good while in the bathroom in the company of a sympathetic nurse, who also cleaned up the bed and the room after me and would not permit me to apologise. She declared that she had dealt with far worse, and that, in any case, it was they, the hospital, that had done this thing to me with their pharmaceutical cocktail!

When my doctor came around later, he took me off all medication. He felt that the rash had been allergic and that, since they didn't know what I had reacted to, it was better to be safe and stop everything. Much later, we discovered that I was, in fact, allergic to the soap powder in which the nursing staff had washed my binder... And in retrospect, the decision to 'stop everything' may not have been very helpful – but it is easy to be wise after the event...

The command the doctor had given meant that I now had no protective cover of any kind against infection. He had made this decision for the very best of reasons. In the circumstances, as far as he could see, it was probably the only sensible course of action. Only with hindsight is it possible to see that this was when things started to go seriously downhill. One by one, I began to experience a range of perplexing problems.

First, an area of the wound at the top of my new left breast opened up, and fluid came from it. All day, I complained that I could smell fried food, just like a chip shop or a Chinese takeaway. The unpleasant truth emerged; it was my own body that I was smelling! The surgeon explained to me that a small part of the grafted fat under the new wound did not have an adequate blood supply and was gradually dying back, becoming liquid. Fat cells were clearly visible in this fluid, and it had a characteristic greasy odour, but it was neither infected, nor particularly offensive. The area that had opened up was to be kept open to allow drainage of this fluid to take place. Eventually, when all the tissue without blood supply was gone, the wound would again heal. So far, so good...but I had no antibiotic protection, and, very soon, the fatty smell was replaced by a foul odour, and I had a staphylococcal infection deep inside that wound. I was also worried because this was already the smaller breast. If tissue inside it was infected, dying and liquefying, this could not be good news!

The wound wept fluid round the clock and had to be dressed with absorbent dressings. Meanwhile, a second wound opened, on the right breast in roughly the same place. This wept a different and bloodstained fluid. On my abdominal wound, two areas turned ominously yellow and sticky. The wound on my navel was becoming rather wet, too.

One of the doctors suggested the nurse use a 'wick' in the wound on the right breast. This meant putting a piece of tape into the wound, leaving the end out to keep the wound open. This tape would then help to draw out the fluid inside the wound. It was important that these wounds did not heal over whilst fluid was being produced deep inside them; this would only serve to seal a problem in.

From that day, the nurses began to pack both breast wounds with tape soaked initially in a fluid called 'Intrasite', which helps wounds to slough dead matter, then later with 'eusol and paraffin', widely used in hospitals to clean up nasty wounds. Daily, wet dressings were taken from my abdomen and navel, and the packing removed from the wounds in both breasts. Any remaining fluid would be squeezed from these wounds with a gentle but firm pressure. Then I was put under the shower on a commode chair to have my wash. After washing, clean wound pads would be put on my tummy and fresh packing into my breast wounds. This ritual, however, did not seem to be promoting healing. Day after day saw no improvement. If anything, things were getting worse…

...And I had another problem. I do not usually become sick after a general anaesthetic, but since the long anaesthetic, and throughout this time, I was queasy a great deal. Some of this was no doubt due to the various medications I had, but I coughed up a great deal of phlegm, particularly in the mornings. Sister said my room sounded like six a.m. on the chest ward. My appetite seemed to have largely deserted me. I could not work up enthusiasm for food as before. I also had a small rough patch in my upper throat from a tube used during my operation. It felt like a crumb of food that was only partially swallowed. This seemed to add to the feeling of sickness and reluctance to tackle food.

In the midst of all this, my poor husband was endeavouring to cook for me daily, and to provide things that would entice me to eat. My friends were also still doing the same. The food carrier provided by one friend became the universal hot food transport system, much to the amusement of the ward. It smelled so nice, wafting in. Martin brought organic lamb, freshly cooked vegetables, hotpots and the like. Sometimes he reheated curries other friends had made for me. Visitors brought fresh fruit salads, or tempted me with small fruit, ready washed.

One day, I was enjoying the company of Martin and three friends, all bearing gifts, at my bedside, when the friend who actually owned the food carrier arrived. She had the pot with her, and it was full to the brim! She hadn't known that I would have company, and I was aghast at how much wonderful Chinese stir-fry she had made and the quantity of noodles she had prepared to go with it. Martin begged some plates and forks from the nursing staff, who were happy and amused to oblige, and it is no exaggeration to say that the contents of that pot fed everyone present, and some of us twice, and there was still food left over – a real 'loaves and fishes' event! There was a party atmosphere around the bed that day, and **was** I glad to have friends to share that enormous pot of food! The nursing staff began to compare the food odours coming from my room with those coming from the catering trolley and draw conclusions...

The dressings ritual eventually became a twice-daily event. This was exhausting, and *so* unpleasant! I could do **that** scene from 'Psycho' all by myself! However carefully the nurses tried to ensure the wounds were clean and empty before I moved to the shower, I managed to end up with water and indescribable other things trickling down my body towards my feet. I would sit on that commode chair with the shower head in my hand, while the nurses would hand me disposable wash cloths and squirt 'Aquasept' antiseptic soap over me, or hand me an antiseptic bar to wash with. I felt the way I guess a leper must feel – as if people didn't want to get too close – and I was totally revolted by my own condition. How could other people be expected to tolerate me if I could not tolerate myself? I winced in disgust and distaste. It seemed no amount of washing would stop the wound on my left breast from smelling.

One night, one of the nurses put a charcoal dressing on it, since I was complaining of the smell right under my nose. As she did this she stated that she was only dressing the wound in this way because she believed in holistic care and wanted me to feel better and not because she felt it was necessary. It seems that, in general, others were not aware of the odour. For me, it was a constant companion. I had been warned by the surgeon that this situation would take a long time to resolve, but I felt it was **not** resolving. I became increasingly sick and increasingly despondent.

At this time, the consultant advised that I should start wearing a bra, to support my breasts through this process of infection and fat necrosis. Fine, but I didn't own any! And how was I going to try anything on, whilst I was in this state? I described my washing sessions as 'gunge-fests'! And anyway, how was I going to **get** bras to try on in the first place?

With the help of a companionable and 'no nonsense' nurse, and a telephone, all was sorted. I phoned a lingerie chain first, but the lady who answered was not sure that they had what I needed and therefore suggested I phone Debenhams, which I did. The staff could not have been more helpful. I explained my circumstances, the nurse measured me around and below the bust line, and the store staff put aside some bras they thought might fit, which my husband collected.

Now all we had to do was to find a way to try these things on hygienically! My practical nurse again came up with the answer, and a very old-fashioned one it was, too!

When I was a child, wanting to help my mother in the kitchen, she would sometimes put one of her pinafores on my front, pulling the neck loop, which of course was much too big, down to my waist at the back, and tying the waist strap through it, thus making the garment shorter. Now my nurse did much the same thing. She tied a plastic apron, such as the staff wear for protection, around me, hitching it up, just as my mother had done so long ago. This meant that the widest part of the apron was around my bust, and all of my wounds and dressings were well covered. This done, we tried on the bras. The one that fitted best was a 36D. Considering that I had asked the surgeon for 'two fried eggs' this was rather a surprise! The bras that didn't fit were returned to the shop unscathed, and two more of the right size purchased. Mission accomplished!

Besides the whole business of the messy wounds, around this time I also began to experience wildly fluctuating temperatures which tended to peak in the evening and caused concern and consternation, since these peaks were often very high. I was really quite ill, so ill that my morning ablutions sometimes seemed to take for ever.

One day, three special friends turned up to see me and I was only in the middle of this process. Weak and weepy, I was very afraid they'd not be able to wait as long as they'd have to. At first they thought that, in that state, visitors might be too much for me, but when they understood me more clearly these great people went off and ate crispy bacon rolls in the cafeteria then returned to spend some time with me once I was done. When you feel as low as I did that day, empathetic friendship like that is so precious, and time is such a special gift!

During this time, I was still being encouraged to walk up and down the ward for exercise. On one occasion, as I was having a wander with Martin at my side, we saw a man sitting in a wheelchair the dayroom, with nothing to stare at but the wall. Since he was still there when we passed again a little while later, we stopped in the doorway to ask if he was O.K. He said that he was, but that his foot, which was bandaged, was very painful. Could we pass a stool to him? I was not allowed to lift anything, but Martin obliged. The man thanked us and we moved on.

Back in my room a little while later, I heard the ward sister on the telephone. It seemed she was trying to find a bed for this patient, who would need to be barrier nursed, since he had MRSA, the superbug antibiotic resistant infection. I had merely spoken to him; I hadn't even entered the room, yet I was so scared! The last thing I wanted was MRSA. I was in enough trouble already. Had Martin touched him, I wanted to know? Martin had no patience with all this. **He** wanted to know where my faith was! After all, he had only done the decent thing by helping this poor chap, and given the situation again, he would help him again. It was the only possible Christian response. He had washed his hands when we returned to my room anyway, so where was the concern? In my head I knew he was right, but still I fretted. So often we put ourselves through hell when we pre-empt a fearful circumstance in this way. We force ourselves to experience a horror that has no place in our lives, just by fearing it. In fact, I hadn't become infected. If I had simply trusted God, I'd have had a much easier time – but in our humanity, that kind of trust doesn't always come easy, and it didn't, on that occasion, to me.

One fearful thing, and then one beautifully reassuring thing… In the midst of all this angst, I received a card from a church friend, a lady who had really been through the mill herself and was a woman of great faith. Inside the card, she had pasted a poem. I do not know where she cut it from, and there was neither a title at the top nor an author's name at the bottom. I have not been able to trace it, though I have tried hard to do so. I can't explain it, but when I read this verse, it was an extremely emotional experience. It was a cloak of assurance that Jesus was with me. It wasn't just the poem; it was the *timing* of its arrival. So often, that is God's grace; He knows when we most need strength or reassurance, and that is precisely when He sends it, no sooner and no later. I give you the verses in full now, below:

Let it go my friend,
Just let it go and never look back.
Let it go my friend.
Let me be the one to put you back on the track.
My friend you can depend on me.

Let it go my friend.
There's nothing you need to be frightened of.
And you know my friend,
In the midst of your pain you'll experience my love.
My friend you can depend on me.

Put your trust in me. I'll guide you all the way.
Why even the blind can see,
And the deaf hear what I say.
Let it go my friend.

Let go of the pain, let go of the hurt.
Time will show you my friend.
But already you know how much you are worth.
My friend
You can depend on me.

I confess that after I read this, I cried a great deal. It effected some kind of inner healing that I am unable to explain. Still, however, the days wore on and I was not well. I was weak and often had a high temperature and low spirits!

Across the hallway from my room was another single room. The patient here, whom I shall call Sue, was also in for breast reconstruction. She was undergoing the same procedure as me, D.I.E.P. flap, but for a single breast lost to cancer, rather than two. I knew that her pain in the days immediately following surgery would be just as awful as mine had been – stomach ache, back ache, soreness upon moving and so on.

One night, I felt particularly bad. One of the nurses came in to help me, so that I would be comfortable enough to sleep. Tearful, I told her that God had been with me so far and He wasn't going to let go now! On hearing her response: 'No, He won't...' I knew that this nurse was a Christian.

I awoke very early next morning and realised that there was a drama going on, involving Sue's room. I could hear the phone at the nurses' station. I heard the staff nurse express her concern to a doctor that Sue's flap was looking dusky...I heard the doctor come and enter the room opposite... I heard him leave, saying he wished he'd known sooner... I knew what this meant. Despite having all the discomfort that I was experiencing, Sue was also facing the agonising disappointment of flap failure: her graft had not taken. For her, there would be no new breast from the surgery.

I felt terrible – for her, not for myself. Then the nursing shift changed, and my friend of the evening before reappeared. 'I prayed for you last night,' she said. I responded, 'I knew you would... But come in, now, and shut the door, because we need to pray...' I cast my eyes towards the door opposite. 'Oh, yes!' she said immediately, and sat upon my bed. We prayed together for Sue, and, though we were from very different Christian traditions, it did not matter at all. We were even able to agree about asking Jesus's mother, Mary, to add her prayers to ours. Then the nurse went off to do her work.

I picked up the T.V. remote, to put on breakfast television, and it was just as if my wrist had been slapped! It was as if the Lord had said something like, 'You have nothing better to do than watch breakfast T.V. and here is a woman going through a dreadful crisis, and you, a Christian, are sitting there! Now, switch off that T.V. and pray!' I did. I prayed for a little while, until it felt O.K. to stop.

Much later, I found out what happened. The consultant, **my** consultant, came to see Sue. He said to her, 'You came in for a new breast, and you'll go out with a new breast...' Though only half of the flap had not taken, the surgical team decided not to make patchwork. Sue was taken back to theatre, where the original flap was removed and replaced with one from a new donor site on her back. An implant was then used to give a profile matching the other breast. Sue seemed pleased with the result. Though she had an abdominal scar that now seemed superfluous, she was grateful for the incidental 'tummy tuck'. She left hospital a while before I did.

Weeks later, we met in the Outpatients' Clinic. Still healing, she, like me, was a bit fed up with the time it was all taking to resolve, but it did us both good to know that the other was still playing the game and, on that day, we commiserated also over the fact that each of us would still, at some point, need further surgery. 'We might meet up in there!' she said.

The whole incident with Sue helped me to see things differently. For a Christian who has, at any rate, **tried** to give their life to God, even being sick in hospital is not just about self. There is a whole world to interact with in that place, and there are lessons to be learnt and there are tasks to complete. I **know** we were meant to pray for Sue that day, which means I was **meant** to be there at that time...

Something else happened that also served to convince me. The male student nurse who had sat in when I was looking at the results of my surgery for the first time was a member of the Jehovah's Witness community. He came in one day, and we chatted at length. He was, he said, convinced that the Witnesses had got it right. He knew I was Roman Catholic, and I told him that I was a member of that church because that was where my heart lay and where I believed God wanted me to be…that faith was a journey, the Christian Church active and dynamic, and that I believed the church to which I belonged was guiding me best, in the way that God wanted me to walk, which was why I remained a member. Had I felt this way about another Christian tradition, I would doubtless have been a member of that one instead!

Despite these obvious differences of opinion, we conversed for a long time, probably over an hour, covering, amicably, a wide range of topics, then he said, 'What about sinners? People like adulterers?'

I asked him what he meant and he explained that, in his church, members were instructed not to speak to such people, not to tolerate them, not to spend time with them. Effectively, they would be cut off. I explained that it was not like that for us. I told him gently that I had personally had the experience of feeling that someone close to me was doing something very wrong; something against God's teaching. (You don't make it to over fifty years of age without experiences of this kind!) At times like these, if I was struggling, I had sought the advice of my priest on how to handle such things. I explained that, for us, the way forward lay in the example Jesus gave. He fraternised with sinners. He ate with sinners. In any case, we are **all** sinners! How can anyone make a decision that another's sin is so great that he or she deserves to be ostracised, without inviting judgement upon oneself? For us, I explained, the only way forward was love. Yes, I would make it gently clear to that person that I felt that what they were doing was seriously wrong, but I would not feel I had the right to judge them! I may hate the sin, but

Helen Gaize

I had a Christian duty to love the sinner. And I do not believe that anyone was ever led to a genuine change of heart by being ostracised! Surely that could only lead to a hardening of hearts all round? I said that I felt that the only real answer was to love for as long as it took – and that might be a very long time! In this matter, at least, he felt that the approach I put forward was right. Who knows where his subsequent thoughts may have led?

Then there was also the young Islamic doctor. He was gentle, earnest and concerned, and I have no idea why it happened, but one day, while he was struggling to get a blood sample from me (the regular 'bleeders' having already visited with their trolley and having failed), I found myself telling him of the goodness of God, and he was agreeing. Astonishingly, and almost involuntarily (I would, in other circumstances, have been too shy), I went on to tell him what a great gift God had given him in his calling as a doctor – even advising him to value it. I do not think I would normally have had such a conversation in such circumstances. To me, it seemed a special moment somehow. I will probably never know why the conversation took place, but it did, and I know that it meant something to him, and there is a rightness about that.

Throughout my stay in hospital, the chaplaincy team was great. I was supported by visits, and I received Holy Communion on Sundays and on Ascension Thursday. For this I was extremely thankful. There was, however, one thing that happened that fairly blew my socks off! I believe God likes to pull a little surprise out of His sleeve every now and again…

I had asked for someone from the team to bring me Communion on the coming Sunday. When they arrived, the nurses asked them to wait outside for a while, as I was still being washed and dressed. Still very sick, and still having open and productive wounds, I could not hurry this process. Whoever was outside kindly agreed to wait.

Eventually, I combed my hair and opened the door for them to enter – but instead, they stood, surprised and rooted, as did I, and then we flew into each other's arms.

For years, I had been part of the music ministry that played for the healing prayer group in Barking. A couple of years before, a lady who was part of the healing team and her gentle husband had left this prayer group, because they had relocated. I did not know their current address; only that they had returned a couple of times, to keep in touch with friends, but had left early on those occasions because it was a long drive home. Now, here was I, in a hospital at some distance from home, and here, at my door, was this husband and wife team! 'Helen!' she shrieked. 'Anne!' I squealed, 'I *so* need healing prayer!' I flew into her arms, as she said, 'You've got it!'

I found out later that there are about ninety people on that chaplaincy team, any one of whom could have brought me Communion on that day. This couple had no idea that I was in this, their local hospital, and I didn't know that they now lived in this locality. They gave me Communion, listened to my story, chatted, prayed over me for healing, left their telephone number in case I needed anything and generally ministered to me in a really comprehensive and loving way, but the very fact of their presence was like a reassurance of God's ongoing care; a sign that He was looking out for me. I felt sure the morning's events were no coincidence, and I could see that some of the hospital staff found the whole thing fairly impressive, too.

Soon after this, I had a day when my stomach seemed particularly painful and bloated. It was very uncomfortable all day, and I told several nurses. 'Wind,' was the general consensus. That evening, as I was showering, the nurse and I were both pleased to note that there were signs of pink, healthy tissue and fresh blood in my chest wounds, surely an indication that things were about to improve? However, as I washed my lower abdomen, the skin surface began to slosh about like the cover on a water bed. I had a fluid collection inside me, and a large one at that.

The doctors were called, came and generally took stock of my situation: open, productive wounds above both new breasts, a weeping wound site where my navel had been, two patches on the abdominal wound which were yellow and sloughing, a fluid collection below that, and an erratic temperature which was often high. I was not in a pretty state. It was, I think, this cumulative catalogue of problems that provoked the next decision. Now, a couple of weeks after my twelve-hour general anaesthetic, I was to go back to theatre to have my wounds cleaned up and re-sutured.

I did not immediately welcome this decision. I was particularly anxious because most of the problem of fat necrosis had been from the new left breast, which had been smaller than the right from the start. I felt that the necrosis problem already meant further tissue loss from that side. If the surgical team was planning to clean up that site, wouldn't this inevitably mean further tissue loss? However, I realised that I had little alternative. It had been suggested to me once already that I would be in danger of further infection the longer I remained in hospital, and that therefore I might be discharged to manage my own wounds at home. I was aghast at this suggestion. I was told I would be amazed at what people could manage. That may be so, but I was looking at a prospect of not only expressing, cleaning and packing badly infected wounds, but doing so directly underneath my own chin, with little prospect of being able to see what I was at! I didn't think I could manage this, and

Martin was adamant that he could not. The surgeon was certain that, left to themselves, these wound sites would resolve, but this would take a long time – we were talking months. I gave consent for the surgical debrading of all the infected wound sites. I was told I would go back to theatre next day.

Early the following morning, I could hear the surgeon on the ward. I waited for him to come to see me, but he did not. However, a conversation about me between him, his team and a nurse took place audibly outside my closed door. This really troubled me. I felt that the nurse had represented me wrongly in what she had said, and I felt that the surgeon should, perhaps, have spoken *to* me, not *about* me. Troubled by these thoughts for some time, I decided not to let them fester any longer, but to ask to speak to a nurse.

When she came, I told her what I had overheard, what I felt I had actually said to the nurses, and the way I felt that had been misinterpreted by the nurse to the surgical team. I also said that I was surprised not to have spoken with my surgeon.

The nurse now explained all of this to me. If a patient speaks to a nurse, to confide an anxiety or express a concern, for example, that nurse then has a duty to that patient to make other nurses on the team aware of this situation at handover. It is to some extent inevitable, then, that the process is a bit like the game of 'Chinese whispers', where a message changes slightly, each time it is passed further along the line. The nurse apologised for any discomfort I had felt upon hearing myself spoken of, but explained that the nursing staff were concerned at all times for the holistic well-being of the patient. They, after all, had a better overview of how the patient was progressing moment by moment than the doctors did. They wanted the doctors to know of the anxieties and concerns of the patient in order to avoid further heartache for them. This was to ensure appropriate routes in treatment and to protect the patient as a human being as well as a surgical subject. Of the surgeon's failure to visit me, she explained that he would not have entered my room that morning because he was about to go to theatre and I was severely infected. He could not risk spreading the infection. For the same reason, I would be last on the day's list. From this incident, I learnt that it is far better to speak up, (calmly and politely, of course), than to 'stew'.

Something else happened that I assume to be a direct result of that conversation. Later that day, there was a tap on my door and the lady who entered explained to me that she was a counsellor. Now, I had been asked if I wished to see a counsellor before, during my stay, and had declined, with a 'What could **she** do?' However, I invited this lady, who was not at all pushy, and was sensitive at all times, to sit. She seemed surprised that I was not expecting her, but we deduced that the nurse I had spoken to had probably felt it was appropriate to call her. She asked if I would like to talk.

I explained to this patient listener how I had come into hospital for what I hoped would be my final breast operation. I told her what I had been told: that I would be in theatre for six and a half hours, in hospital for seven to ten days, and off work for six weeks, and how different I felt the reality was turning out to be. I told her that I was anxious because I could see that the result of my surgery was uneven. I had one breast bigger than the other. I showed her my chest. We agreed that there was an appreciable difference, and discussed whether it might be rectified by wearing the right bra, or would need more intervention. I told her how frightening and disappointing it had been to have so many problems with infection, even though I had been warned that it could be a complication following the surgery, and I told her of the surgeon's conversation outside my door that morning, and his failure to visit me.

She listened carefully to all that I poured out and then asked me what it was that I would have particularly wanted to talk to the surgeon about. I explained that I was very worried that, after the surgery, the left breast would be even smaller. If the surgeon was also planning to remove infected tissue from the right breast, could he not also take away a little more at the same time, to 'even me up'?

This counsellor was really helpful. She said she very much understood my disappointment and my fears. She felt that my feelings were justified. She also felt that it was very important for me to speak to the surgeon before I was anaesthetised, and she promised, before she left, that she would make sure that I would have a chance to do so. She gave me her card, so that I could contact her again if I felt the need.

The anaesthetist came to see me, a different gentleman from the last time; South African, interested and concerned. (Alas, I remember little of the anaesthetist or the theatre reception team from the first surgery, though I know they were gentle and kind, and I think that is because of the twelve-hour general anaesthetic.) He asked me about how I respond to anaesthetics, and I told him that I had experienced sickness the last time around, though never before. He said he could put something in when mixing my anaesthetic to address that. He really seemed very attentive. After we had dealt with the business he had called to speak about – the GA, my rotten veins, and all that – he said to me, 'Helen, I've got to ask you, is it worth it?'

I had real difficulty with that one. In the end, I said that it was too soon to be able to make a judgement, but I hoped so. I wanted to know why he had asked the question. He explained that he felt it was necessary to treat the whole patient, not just administer an anaesthetic, and clearly I had been through so much. He was right about that one! I explained how I felt about 'self assembly' and that I hadn't worn prostheses, and he said that he felt that the surgical option was always better, because he was sure the alternative must become tedious, long term. He was genuinely interested, and it became clear that he would talk in this way to all his patients, to enable him to empathise more closely with their situations.

I was washed, but not dressed for theatre, when they came for me, as the nurses had told me it wouldn't take a minute to put my gown on and 'do a last wee' when called for. The lady from theatre didn't seem amused, but the frost melted when she saw me make an appropriate effort, and soon we were off.

I don't like that ride on the bed to the theatre. Looking at the ceiling, whilst wildly cornering as corridors meet, very quickly makes me feel seasick. They let me keep my specs, which helped, and promised to label them and be sure I got them back afterwards.

The counsellor had been as good as her word. I was able to speak to the surgeon before the operation. He was understanding but could only reassure me a little. He didn't think I'd lose much more of the left breast tissue, but there was no way that he could remove any tissue from the right side or do any reshaping: 'We are going to remove the infection. If I try to do anything else, I will only spread it.' With that, I had to be content.

In pre-op. there were the usual problems. It proved impossible to find a decent vein in order to get a line in, and many attempts were made. Machinery around me was beeping clinically, and one of the doctors ordered that 'the noise' be turned off to avoid further stress for me. They were very understanding, but I ended up with a line in my left arm. This is never supposed to happen, as I have no lymph nodes on that side to protect me. (There should be plenty in the armpit, but I had had all fifteen of mine removed, and five had been cancerous.) This means that I am always at greater risk of infection if any lines go in on that side and wasn't infection what I had come to theatre to deal with? I was assured that as soon as I was asleep, the line would be re-sited.

About two hours later, I woke up groggily in post-op. After a wait, I was wheeled back to the ward. I discovered that the infected area under the flap forming my left breast had been thoroughly cleaned out, and the flap had been re-sutured at the top, into a different position. A major part of the problems I'd been having, it seemed, was due to the fact that the irradiated skin on the left side of my chest had very poor healing qualities. This is one of the known legacies of radiotherapy. The skin from my stomach, of course, was fine, but it had to heal to the skin native to the chest area, hence the problem. The surgeons hoped that the new suture line they had now created, higher up my chest, would heal better. There was a good chance that part of me had received less radiation and the skin from my tummy would be able to bond to it as it should.

Wounds had also been cleaned and re-sutured in my right breast, my navel, and in a goodly part of the abdominal scar. The fact that I had been re-stitched was a very good sign, apparently. The nurses told me that if the doctors had felt there was a risk of the wounds remaining infected despite the surgery (and therefore continuing to be productive), they would have sent me back from theatre with the wounds cleaned, but open to allow drainage. There were, however, a couple of 'downsides', too…

The sutures put in during the original surgery had been soluble and beautifully fine, leaving very little scarring. Being soluble, they did not last more than a few weeks. The surgeons had felt that, since my healing ability, especially on irradiated sites, seemed poor, I would need stronger stitches this time, which could be left in place longer, to support the flesh whilst it healed. These stitches would obviously create much more definite scarring, but they were necessary, and that was that. Also, the re-siting of the top line of my left breast flap had served to slightly flatten the profile of this already smaller breast. It was going to take more than the right bra to sort this out!

I had now been on the receiving end of three trips to theatre. Knowing how I felt about receiving blood, the team had not transfused me, but the issue of transfusion now became a daily, sometimes it seemed an hourly, subject for discussion. I had lost a fair quantity of blood. I had not eaten as well as I usually did, partly due to the complication over diet, and partly due to nausea. My Hb (haemoglobin – with iron needed to carry oxygen) was down to 7.9. A healthy Hb is around 12. Sometimes, people suffer a gradual drop in Hb over a period of time due, for example, to poor diet. Such people often function normally, even with a very low count, because their bodies have had time to adjust. However, a sudden and distinct drop, such as mine, can lead to breathlessness, fainting, light-headedness, poor ability to heal – a host of potential problems. Every time I saw the consultant, it seemed transfusion was mentioned.

I remained very fearful about this prospect, despite prayer and counsel. I was taking iron tablets. I had been taking them since just after the first surgery. Surely my Hb would soon start to climb? I ate iron rich foods. Martin brought me organic eggs and spinach in quantities. In short, I did everything in my power to improve my situation, but my count stubbornly remained at around 8 despite it all. I spoke to the nurses. They felt that a transfusion might be necessary, but, with typical honesty, admitted they wouldn't want it themselves. One movingly described how transfusions that she had feared had saved the life of her child. I spoke to family members, too. And I remained very afraid of transfusion. Meanwhile, with my veins always a problem, and my body now bruised all over, it became more and more difficult to obtain the necessary samples for blood tests. The day came when the surgeon said, 'If you stay here, you will definitely get MRSA. I cannot send you home as anaemic as this. If your Hb is less than 9 tomorrow, we are going to transfuse you.'

That night I hardly slept. I spoke to any nurse who would listen and then, knowing both to be 'night owls' I called first my husband, then my father – the latter at two a.m.! What should I do? The hospital staff could not force me to receive a transfusion, but I did not want to compromise my recovery, much less to catch MRSA. Still uneasy, with the aid of those who advised me, I reached a decision: I would be guided by the surgeon's advice.

Don't ask me to explain, because I can't, but the prospect of receiving blood *so* scared me, still. In my mind, I saw the point when the first few drops had entered my circulation and there would be no going back, and no way to get it out. And yet I had been a blood donor, and I would have wanted my own donated blood to be valued, not feared. I prayed, I sought reassurance from the Bible and received several passages assuring me of the Lord's unceasing care for me, and in the end, dozed off.

Next day, not one word was said by the surgeon about transfusion! And, I discovered something else that was profoundly moving.

The friend who plays lead guitar in the music ministry that I belong to had offered to give **his** blood, being a universal donor, in the hope that I might feel more secure in accepting such help. In the end, I knew this to be impractical, due to the time that would be taken in mandatory screening, but what a touching gesture that was! And how blessed am I, once again, in my friends? Indeed, I think that it was mainly due to friends and family that I made it through that period with my sanity intact! God, in His goodness, saw to it that I had tremendous support from my visitors. I even received a visit from my father, who lived at a great distance in the Midlands. My thoughtful sister and her husband kindly picked him up and brought him. It was such a tonic to see them all when I was feeling so low. Sometimes, though we may not recognise it ourselves, God knows that the medicine we need is love, not drugs, and He sends it in large doses to our bedsides!

My Hb never climbed above 8 whilst I was on the ward, but I never was transfused. I was told that, to protect me from further exposure to infection, I needed to go home, but that, anaemic as I was, I'd have to arrange to have company around the clock, at least to begin with, in case I fainted, and, in falling, damaged a wound site or my flaps. I telephoned a few of my closest friends, who, between them, arranged a 'Helen sitting' rota, because poor Martin, who had arranged time to be with me for the week after surgery and the first week at home, had long since had to return to work, since his wife's 'week' in hospital had become twenty two days! I **was** going home!

I tried to thank my surgeon before leaving the hospital, but he would not accept my thanks. I think he felt as disappointed as I did at the way things had turned out for me. He told me to save my gratitude for later, when all would be healed and finished. I felt it was an awkward conversation. Drugs were sent up from the pharmacy for me to take home with me – I would still be on a cocktail of antibiotics for a long time – and I packed up my possessions ready to leave. In twenty-two days, you accumulate a great deal in a hospital room! I had asked Martin to bring in some treats with which to thank the staff, which he did, and then we said our goodbyes and left – slowly – because I was still very weak and unsteady.

It seemed to be a strange 'half-life' that I returned to. My friends were as good as their words and there was someone with me whenever Martin was out on business, save for very short periods. These times of companionship were precious for the sharing, the counsel and sometimes the prayer times together that they afforded. I quizzed my companions endlessly because I knew that, after all I had been through, the result of my surgery was very uneven and I found it hard to cope with this in any way. I had consented to this whole procedure seeking symmetry above all. Now, if I dressed carefully, there were some clothes in which the lack of balance did not show, but I was extremely unhappy to have gone through so much and, after it all, to be as obviously uneven in the chest area as I then was.

The thing that made me most unhappy was the prospect of having to use some form of prosthesis in my bra to level things up. I had said long before that I was 'through with self-assembly'. That had been the main reason I had been so determined to go through with the second mastectomy, after which I had just thrown on a crop top and got on with my day – with an attitude of 'what you see is what you get'. Now I knew that the difference between my new breasts was too great to pass unnoticed and I hated the thought of having to wear a partial prosthesis – with a passion!

I also knew, though it took me a very long time to admit that I knew it, that I was going to have to go back for further surgery. This was something I fought against acknowledging: I had been afraid of the risks of surgery the last time – and it had been elective, not life-saving. Could I contemplate it again?

A good friend spent an afternoon with me whilst I was, frankly, in the depths of a depression induced by all this, and she, always a no-nonsense character, talked a lot of her good sense into me. If I needed to 'do something' to make me look normal in a bra, then I would do it. That way, I would look unremarkable and would resume my life. Shortly afterwards, I went to the tallboy drawer in my bedroom and found four small foam bust enhancing cups that I had used about three times in all since choosing to go 'flat', in order to give a little definition to my shape in certain clothes. Essentially, they were circles of foam covered in flesh-coloured nylon, with a small segment of the circle cut out to give a slightly conical shape. I experimented with inserting one of these into the bra cup on my 'deficient' side and found that the look thus created was more than adequate to pass muster – but it was still a form of the hated 'self-assembly'…

This may sound crazy if you've never been there, but this is how I got around it: somehow I felt, and I urge you to try this if it applies to 'where you're at' that if the bust cup was **part** of the bra it wouldn't matter so much – maybe because I'd be back to being able to 'throw it on and go' – I don't know. Anyhow, I had four bras, bought when I was in the hospital and the surgeon said that the healing breasts needed support, and two pairs of these bust cups, so I set to with a needle and thread and stitched the bust cups loosely into the left cup of each bra, anchoring them at three points only, so as to ensure that the modification was not visible from the front of the bra – and it worked. Once dressed, I looked absolutely normal, and, somehow, because they were now integral with the bras, it did not feel as if I was assembling myself rather than dressing: it was O.K.

The other thing took longer. I had a huge question mark in my head as to what to do about my shape. One day, in the depths of depression, I telephoned my father. I wept down the phone to him about how I felt that I had merely exchanged one form of deformity for another, and, since the surgery had been elective, how I had to admit that I had done this thing to myself. I had gone through so much and, I felt, achieved so little – and I was so sad about it all. He was helpless as to how to respond. In the end, sensing that I might not somehow be giving him a balanced view, I put my friend, who was present, on to talk to him, and listened in a half-hearted way to her more positive version of things.

Something rather strange was happening here. My surgeon had achieved a remarkably good result, given the devastation of my chest. What he had achieved, in the twelve gruelling hours of microsurgery, was little short of miraculous. Yet at this point, I was truly unable to see that, for all the surgical skill that had been used on me, I had gained anything. I hated the unevenness of my new breasts, thought myself hideous and was unable to see that the position I was then in was any better, really, than where I was at before the operation. It was true that I still had some pretty hideous lesions on the 'seam lines' of my new breasts. Although I was now at home, there was a dressings ritual to be got through, initially twice a day, then later daily. This involved a great deal of care for fear of the danger of further infection. Martin and I went through the whole thing together, keeping a close watch on each other for any breach in the hygiene of how we were tackling this. Dressings were at this time very soiled and the wounds were still quite large. One was the size and shape of a human eye, and so deep that the bottom of it could not be seen. The old dressings had to be removed, and any secretions expressed from the wounds. I had to shower, using a bactericidal soap, being very careful not to contaminate open lesions with, for example, a sponge that might have touched other insalubrious body parts, and I had then to place clean gauzes over the wound sites, but dry the rest of my body on a towel. Iodine impregnated dressings (Inadine patches) were then applied, followed by gauze swabs or a wound pad to absorb the inevitable secretions, then adhesive dressings keeping the lot in place, and a clean bra for support. To be honest, it was all pretty vile. Small wonder, then, that I was depressed.

My father and my friends tried to talk me round. My closest friend became increasingly frustrated because she felt that I misinterpreted everything she said to me. I don't know about this. In any conversation, one can never be sure that what one says is necessarily what the other person hears. Because the words have to be processed through the brain of the listener, they **will** be 'flavoured' before being interpreted. Perhaps this explains the problems of communication we had at this time. I only know that I felt *so* down – and so let down by all that had happened to me: it wasn't supposed to be like this!

My aunt, my father's sister, spoke at length to me over the phone and told me that *she* was not a bit surprised – she had expected this from the moment I had described the procedure to her. She spoke of how her brother, my uncle, had been advised that he would need one or two operations, which had in fact turned out to be eight! Though these revelations had some comforting aspects to them, I was in some kind of limbo, and that is where the photographs came in...

Before I had gone into hospital, remember, I had begged Martin to take photographs of my chest with the digital camera. I had actually said at the time (and later forgotten) that I wanted them for when I began to wonder why I did this thing to myself. The hospital had sent me to Medical Photography before the operation, but I never saw *those* photographs (though nowadays I have them on disc, having requested them from Medical Records). Now, at my request, Martin printed the ones that he had taken. I *so* needed to see those pictures…and when I did, I realised how faulty my memory was…and maybe my perspective, too…

Partly, I guess, it was the fact that I usually saw my chest from looking down at it; this is not the way that it is seen by others or, in fact, the camera…

Looking at these photographs, I was looking at a scene of real devastation. My chest did not appear just flat-ish, with bumpy scarring, in these photographs, but very irregular indeed. The left side had a large pit, going down through the site of my missing pectoral muscle, to the ribs, which were visible under a paper-thin layer of skin. The side of the chest next to my arm had a lump of skin missing, as if a bite had been taken out. On the right side, the body fat that had been retained had, in part, formed itself into a bolster along the lower bra-line. Thus I had a flat surface to the right chest wall, but with a higher profile than the left, sporting a scar like a gash, and with a 'bolster' underneath it…NOT pretty!

Boy, did it do me good to see those pictures! OK, I had a very odd chest after the surgery, with a right breast a great deal bigger than the left, but my ribs were not on display, and, aside from the wounds, which would eventually heal, there were no holes. At last I was able to say that yes, I had gained something from the surgery. I did not look right, but I did look so much better. This was something my friends and my husband had been telling me all along. They had been puzzled that I did not believe the current situation to be better than before. How could it be, they asked, that I could not *see* that things were better now? How could **anybody** not see…? And, seeing the photographs, I believe my emotions began to heal. O.K., we were not 'home free', but we *were*, undeniably, a step along the way… Also, I began to admit to myself, if I needed more surgery, I may just have to go forward in faith. After all, if you put yourself into the hands of God to do something that you feel is right and that you are led to do, there is no point at all in withdrawing that hand just because things didn't happen in the way you expected them to – God is still God, and the goal is still the goal…and in the end, His way of working is bound to be best.

The tedious discipline of the dressings seemed to govern life for a while, as did the need to sit a great deal and eat a lot of foods rich in iron whilst popping pills that upset my stomach and made me feel sick. I have never been a great meat eater, but I actually developed a taste for organic lamb's liver, and seemed also to be eating spinach with everything.

Meanwhile, I had to attend the dressings clinic at the hospital regularly so that they could monitor my progress. Here, as mentioned before, I met Sue who had been with me on the ward – the one whose initial surgery had been unsuccessful due to flap failure. She was, as I noted earlier, rather down because she was not yet healed and I believe it did us both good to know there was someone else in the same boat. Each of us was coming away clutching a bulging plastic bag full of bulky dressings, so that mentally we were able to make comparisons as we studied these, and feel the fellowship they bestowed!

On these visits to the dressings clinic, I was so afraid of picking up yet more infections that I must have seemed very difficult to the nurses, at least one of whom resorted to allowing me to sanitize my own hands and help! There was, for me, a constant sense of being at risk and ending up with yet more to deal with...

Speaking of 'more to deal with', there were a couple of occasions when events did take a turn for the worse. The first was the night when I discovered I had a spreading red patch above the wound at the top of the new right breast...It seemed to be tracking across the suture line from my surgery, but also flaring up towards my neck, and it looked angry. I was advised to return to the hospital, where I was seen by one of the surgeons involved in my initial and subsequent operations. This was such a relief because he knew me well and knew my case. It wasn't like being seen by a duty doctor who was not conversant with my situation.

The doctor tried to express fluid from the breast, feeling sure that there was a collection in there, but achieved nothing and had to give up. He cleaned my wounds once more, cutting away dead tissue, and then sent me home with instructions to return the next day to see the consultant, and the reassurance that, as far as he could see, the open wound sites themselves were not infected.

The following day things looked better, perhaps due to the cleansing of the wounds, and the consultant determined that the spreading redness would, in all likelihood, 'sort itself out' – Well thank God! – No more nasty intravenous antibiotics! We returned home relieved...

Then came the evening when I was, for a short time, alone in the house, Martin having gone out in the car to collect our son. I had been disturbed, earlier in the evening, to discover a bump in the skin, a bit like a blister in shape, but not as thin, along the wound line at the top of my right breast. It was ugly, I felt, and disfiguring, and I had enough ugly and disfiguring features to deal with. I spoke on the phone to my dad about it and he suggested it might be a feature of a wound that is healing by granulation, from the bottom. He had once had a wound that had behaved this way, on his foot. I spoke also to my closest friend – a nurse, remember – who told me this was 'a small thing' and that I really must stop allowing myself to become upset over little things like this and recognise what was really important…

With Martin gone, I was taking a shower, so had cleaned my wound sites before beginning, and as I climbed out, having applied gauze to the appropriate places, I dabbed myself dry. I walked into the bedroom and saw gleaming wetness on the top of my right breast, which I *knew* I had dried. It was about where that raised lump had been – the one I had noticed earlier. Gently, I pressed the breast and amber coloured liquid came… and came…and came. But by this time, I was armed. I had seen this before. 'This,' I said to myself, 'is our old friend fat necrosis, and I've learnt how to tackle it.' Unphased, I went into battle!

From our heap of dressings I drew out packs of sterile gauze swabs. I think I went through about eight packs of six swabs each, gently expressing the warm amber fluid from a pinprick burst in the 'seam' above my breast. With each application of pressure, the fluid escaped from the pinhole until, finally, the flow ceased. I dressed the little wound with a sterile covering, then telephoned the ward. By now it was around midnight. 'Is there,' I asked, 'anybody there who remembers me?' The immediate reply was 'I should think so, Helen!' then the nurse gave her name, and it was the very same one with whom I had prayed when in hospital. She sought advice for me, and it was decided that I should not wait for my next appointment at the dressing clinic, but should attend the hospital in the morning.

Arriving bright and early, I told my tale. I was seen by a nurse who knew me – she had recently taken out stitches for me – and she called for a doctor. The one who came was a young lady I had regularly seen on the ward; on one occasion she had prescribed antibiotics for me. **She** determined that I needed to be seen by a member of the team who had performed my surgery, so a call went out, and down came the young doctor who had assisted, and who had cleaned my wounds for me on my recent night-time visit. Considering the number of hospital staff and the logistics of shifts and theatres, I feel that this sequence of events was nothing short of a miracle!

The doctor watched as I expressed a little fluid for his benefit, agreed my diagnosis, and said that he felt there was little left for him to do – I had already dealt with the major part of the problem. I reminded him that he had been convinced that there was a fluid collection in the breast, and that his judgement was now vindicated. He said, 'I **knew** there was a collection there!' He enlarged the pinhole with surgical scissors, so that the wound could drain more freely, injecting me with local anaesthetic before cutting, and once more cleaned my wounds, remarking that, by all appearances now, they would soon be healed. He advised me to buy some Betadine, and to keep the wound he had made open by pushing in the point of a gauze pad soaked in this iodine liquid, before dressing the site. Finished, he put on a really large absorbent dressing, for me to go home. 'But it's my **big** side!' I wailed. However, I dressed, and, as I was leaving, he remarked, 'Actually, it gives quite a nice shape!'

Between and alongside my minor medical/surgical crises, I was also attending physiotherapy sessions at regular intervals.

These were extremely reassuring, because I had found the long periods of inactivity very difficult – indeed they had made me twitchy and I felt they may have been responsible for the terrible episodes of 'restless legs' that I had suffered when in hospital, particularly during my enforced bed-rest, which had caused me to resort to drinking large quantities of tonic water as a remedy.

Physio sessions were, however, hardly challenging. The therapist would say something like, 'How far can you raise your right arm? How near can you get it to the side of your head?' and I would raise my arm until it was resting against my ear… Apparently, I was making rapid progress. This, they said, was because I had been a regular at the gym before the surgery. Such conscientiousness is not, it is felt, helpful to the surgery itself, but it pays huge dividends in the recovery period.

The greatest benefit by far that I received from the physio sessions was, without doubt, the reassurance that I spoke of. Remember, I had had it drummed into me that there were certain movements I **must not** make until given permission, for fear of threatening the survival of my flaps, so I would check things out and ask questions constantly. It was great to be told I was on the right track and that it was now safe to raise an arm above a certain point or lift such and such an object, for example. It was also good to be advised on how to help my scars by massaging them, and how to feel connected to my totally numb tummy by exercising it, so that, unable to feel anything at the surface of the skin, I could still feel the muscular movement of the 'crunches' underneath!

Now, I began to feel the need to resume my old life, and, still wearing dressings, returned part time to school. My colleagues had been nothing short of fantastic. They had visited me at home, bearing gifts – and *what* gifts! An enormous datura tree with angel trumpet flowers, and…a necklace of pink pearls with matching earrings! The pearls just don't stop coming, and every time, it seems it is God's reassurance that He hasn't forgotten His promise to bring good things out of the situation that began with my diagnosis of breast cancer. Apparently, my friends had looked for pearls specifically, knowing that they had a special meaning for me. I was really touched by their kindness. Now I was easing my way back into this, my working environment, and I was surrounded by love and support. Even friends and colleagues from my previous workplace made the effort to check on my progress and uphold me with their calls and good wishes. Things like that are the real blessings in this life…

Before the surgery, a colleague who has become a particular friend had said, 'I hope you don't mind, but I'd like to suggest that, after this surgery, you let your hair grow. You have remarked several times on how nice other people's hair looks, and I think it would do you good to have a more feminine image.' Following this, I had brought in a picture from 'before' to show her the long hair I used to have, until chemotherapy made the change necessary. She had greatly admired that photograph. In something of a quandary now, because some of my musical friends, and one in particular, had near enough *forbidden* me to return to my long hair, I decided to let it grow a little; to have a slightly softer image. After living with this for a while, I would see what transpired.

It was so good to be back, but I tired easily. It took me two weeks to get up to speed, during which everybody was incredibly patient, and, just as it seemed I was maybe back into the swing, we broke up for the summer! Maybe this was God's timing. I could have quality healing time to regroup inside my head…

The summer break brought its own challenges. I needed to make the effort to get fit once more. I therefore contacted the ever-patient young athlete who had been my trainer and advisor, following my G.P. referral to the gym. She had gone private and no longer worked there, but I was happy to pay for an hour of her time in order to set up a rehabilitative programme.

She was, as ever, great, and worked it all out for me, so I returned to more vigorous exercise. (Since leaving the hospital, I had been encouraged to walk, daily if possible, and a little further each time than the last. As the anaemia came under control, I had been faithful about this, such that Martin was heard to remark that it was all very well going a little further each day, but if we weren't careful we might end up at John O' Groats!) Anyhow, returning to the gym felt good, though I no longer believed, as one doctor had long ago tried to tell me, that it would really improve my appearance by developing muscle. How could he have said that to me, if he knew the very muscle I would need to develop had been surgically removed? Told me that I could perhaps, with work, have a five, but never a six-pack? Maybe he was just green and inexperienced and he *didn't* know, or maybe he just couldn't face where I was at any more than I could, and risked giving me false hope – who knows? Either way, I had, since then, bitten the bullet and had gone at least part of the way to a surgical solution. Now I was working out again, and, with my little bit of foam in my bra, looked unremarkable. I felt better for it.

I wasn't the only one to note that I felt better! I had a hospital appointment early in the summer break, at which my surgeon announced that, since I had, after all, recovered so well, it was time to consider my situation. He wanted to know how I felt about my uneven boobs.

I had prayed about this moment for some time; 'Lord, when I have to make a further decision about surgery, let me make the *right* one.' Suddenly the moment was here, and I didn't even think about it; I told the surgeon I thought they needed correction at the same time as he told me much the same thing, but then he took my breath away, by suggesting I return to the hospital in September. All previous talk around this subject had been pointing more towards nothing happening before Christmas time, if indeed it was happening at all. I remonstrated. What about my job? Couldn't it be done in the holidays? However, the holidays are, apparently, reserved for children who need to avoid missing further time off school, and I, as a teacher, could understand that. I told them to send me a date and I'd see what I could do. Then we went home and I phoned my head teacher, reluctant to disturb her vacation, but still more reluctant to spring this on her at the start of the new school year. To her credit, she was very reasonable. We could do nothing more about it at this point. Time to get on with life and enjoy the sunshine!

The other perk of the summer, of course, is holidays. We had not dared to make plans and now time was tight. And I did not want to go too far from home in case of any kind of medical problem cropping up. After much research on the Teletext and the Internet, we found a lovely little bed-and-breakfast in Mevagissey, Cornwall. Martin and I asked Dan, our son, if he wished to come with us (he was still then living at home) but he declined, so we booked, just the two of us, having only to please ourselves, and what a luxury that was!

Have you noticed that nothing ever seems to go quite that smoothly? We had arranged our holiday to follow our children's birthdays, which fall close together in August. This year there was to be a special celebration for Dan's twenty-first. He chose a lovely restaurant in London, at Canary Wharf, and we booked for just the four of us, at his request. I managed to ring the restaurant on the quiet and arrange for a birthday cake with the names of both of our children on it, and we had a wonderful evening, eating out by the water and under the stars. It was so good to be together like that.

When we returned home, there was a message on the answerphone: please could we ring the tiler? Now, we had been living with a problem floor for ten years or thereabouts. The previous owners of our house had had an extension built rather cheaply. The floor level in this extension had always been lower than that of the room it adjoined, and whilst the extension sported a tiled floor in grey, chipped vinyl, that in the adjoining room was chocolate brown...*and* there was a great crack across the floor where the extension had fallen away, due to subsidence, over which we had to put a room divider and a doormat. Do you get the less than wonderful picture?

Well, we had taken a quote from a neighbour with a great reputation for his tiling job, and had accepted that quote, and it was this same person who wanted us to contact him. Due to leave for our holiday on the coming weekend, I rang him the next morning, the Tuesday, and he said, 'Basically, I can start tomorrow or not until October.' I asked how long the job would take, and explained our situation, and he said he *thought* we'd be finished by the time Martin and I would need to leave...

This was mid-August. It was, in fact, the very week that I was first officially allowed to lift anything of weight, following my surgery, and I had two rooms to clear by morning – And, moreover, poor Martin, already at work when I made this executive decision, didn't know yet what was about to hit him! Now, I'm not saying it was the wisest move, but something had to be done, and done quickly, so I set about emptying cupboards and spreading their contents around the house, hopefully in such a way as to cause minimum disruption to life while the floor was being remedied. I did have willing assistance from our son when it came to carrying oak dining chairs up the stairs, but let's just say it wasn't a convalescent day!

Martin arrived home in trepidation, having had a phone-call from me. He wasn't looking forward to trying to lift my grandma's oak dresser, but he knew it would have to be done! In the event, it was friends to the rescue once more; May, my Malaysian friend, dropped by, phoned her son, and called in the troops, and soon the rooms were empty…and the house didn't look *too* bad…

True to his promise, our neighbour and his team began work next day, removing old and broken tiles, chiselling out and fixing the crack in the floor, levelling two floors into one and making a superb job of the tiling. After waiting so long, it was just wonderful to see this happen. Without the room divider, the light just flooded in, and what a difference it made! In addition, they finished the job the day before we were due to depart, so we even had time to move a few things back in.

So much for being able to get back to 'working out'. I tell you, moving out of, and back into, two rooms, with the accumulated stuff of years, beats any gym session hollow and then some, but we did it, and now we really could take a vacation – and we really needed to!

Before we set off, I stitched two more of my 'little foam friends' into the left cups of my two swimming costumes. That way I was ready for anything. However, having threatened to be the hottest summer on record, the weather now turned, becoming much more moderate, so, rather than sea bathing, we in fact looked to other pursuits.

The vacation, only six days in all, began with a flying overnight visit to my cousin in Southampton, someone I have always thought of as a big (elder) brother, my own dear brother being younger (though wiser!) than me. Mart and I stayed in the greatest of comfort and were royally entertained and organically fed, because, bless my cousin's dear heart, he had been ringing round the family doing research on what I could and couldn't eat. It was with reluctance that we left the following day, bidding farewell to our hosts, one human and two Airedale canines.

The B 'n B was all we'd hoped for and more. We had a lovely comfortable room (twin beds, but there's more than one way to skin a cat...) with a sea view and beautifully clean en-suite facilities. The breakfasts were great, and, once they'd realised I couldn't eat the bacon and sausages, we settled into a very satisfying 'egg and grilled tomatoes' routine that suited me very well, with grapefruit to start and tea with soya milk to finish. Martin, of course, smelling good bacon frying, was delighted to have the opportunity for a very inviting full English breakfast and made the most of it, and who can blame him?

Every day was different and we were able to do so much that we had wanted to do. We visited the Eden Project and the Lost Gardens of Heligan. We attended a country fair, and watched shire-horses parade. We toured Goonhilly Earth Station, and to my surprise I was absolutely fascinated; we were there about four hours, and when we finally left, it was to go and watch the seals play off Lizard Point as the sun slowly disappeared. We also visited a centre for alternative energy with windmills generating the electricity, and a clay quarry, which was still being worked, and we spent a lot of time on Bodmin Moor, and walked to the standing stones known as 'The Hurlers'.

This was altogether a healing time: we had quality time to spend together and no pressures. Each evening we could decide where to eat and what time to turn in, and I had a little time too for my guitar each day. Maybe it was because I had been denied the opportunity to play for a long time (following the surgery) that this mattered to me. We revelled in each other's company, and talked a great deal in a companionable and easy way. I was letting go of the stress of the surgery and Martin was at last laying aside some of the whopping burden of pressures and responsibility that it had stacked on his shoulders. Altogether, the vacation was a blessing in many ways. God is good!

Once we were back in Harlow, life hit us again with a bit of a bang. I received a letter from the hospital, giving the proposed date of the corrective surgery. It was just three weeks into the new school term. This meant that, as soon as I returned to work, I had to begin the business of finding people to cover for me, and setting cover work for my students. The last is a task that I always find very difficult, because I don't believe in students marking time with tasks intended to keep them busy until the teacher returns. What is set for them must be relevant and appropriate and continue the pace of their education, so the task is very intense and time consuming – Yet all the time, there is the possibility that the hospital will cancel and the set work become irrelevant, despite the hours spent in putting it in place.

People were once more universally very kind, and many happily offered cover. Some, unaware of the 'foam friends' I had been sporting, wanted to know why I had to go back in, but I was forthright about what had to be done and listeners were sympathetic. Even my students were quite reasonable about the whole thing, though I spared them the details! I had been told that, this time, I'd probably be three days in hospital and then need two weeks off. I set work for this period, and left school the day before my admission.

My family was also very supportive. My brother and his wife, over on a visit from New Zealand, had no doubt of the wisdom of 'getting things sorted out', nor did my father, my sister, ('Yes, you do need sorting,') my cousins or my daughter. My husband understood perfectly and upheld me in every way, particularly with his constant reassurance that I was doing the right thing, would not die under anaesthetic in some dreadful accident, and would not succumb to MRSA.

My aunt, however, was very concerned, did not want me to take the risk, questioned my return to hospital if I was no longer as radically disfigured as I had been at first, and asked me why I was *prepared* to risk it. I offered to show her my chest, so that she would be able to understand better, but she declined. Her concern for me was deep and genuine, and she told me of a hospital ward she had been on where every patient caught MRSA. I believe that, to her, this was essentially cosmetic surgery and it made no sense for me to be willing to take what she saw as being a huge risk. All of this negative talk only served to put me in need of a great many further reassurances from poor Martin, who must have felt like a vinyl record with a scratch on it!

A strange thing happened at this time of deep concern. Since the early days of my cancer, I had received the same scripture text from Jeremiah a number of times from different sources. By now, I had very much made it mine, for I found it to be a great source of encouragement. Reading the novel that was my current companion on the day before admission or thereabouts, the scripture popped out of the page in front of me! There it was again: 'I know the plans I have for you, says the Lord... Plans to give you hope and a future'...

I gained reassurance from another source too, for the night before I was due to be admitted to hospital, I went with a group of close friends to the Barking prayer group where we had so long been part of the music ministry. I had been away for a long time, partly due to the long convalescence from my previous surgery, and partly due to the commitments of others in the music group. I filled them in on what had been happening to me, and they prayed over me and for me. Such covering grace is invaluable.

Having phoned the specified ward before nine in the morning as requested, to check that there was a bed available for me, I was due to be admitted on Wednesday for surgery on Thursday. From the start things did not go as planned, but we had prayed about this thing, so I decided that the hand of God was in it, and I'd go with the flow. He was in charge.

Arriving at the designated ward, the one where I'd undergone my previous surgery, I was asked to wait in the dayroom. After a while, a nurse came to say that, in fact, there was no bed available on Iris Ward, so I'd need to be transferred to Jonquil. Assured that I'd still be under the same consultant, we duly trooped round to Jonquil, only to be told there'd been a mistake, and I should be on Marguerite Ward, so off we set again.

Once there, I was allocated a bed, seen by a member of my consultant's team, a junior doctor, and told that I'd be nil by mouth from midnight, and second on my consultant's theatre list in the morning.

Later I was told that actually a different consultant would operate, and he then came to see me. It had been decided to improve my symmetry by reducing the larger breast, since I did not want the smaller augmented with an implant, having long-ago stated that I wanted nothing but my own body tissues in there… The consultant said that he would err on the side of caution with my surgery, for fear of removing too much tissue and I asked him not to be *too* cautious, saying that I didn't want to make a return visit. I told him I would place myself in his hands and in God's and he responded by saying that we are all in God's hands. I liked him. I liked my usual consultant as well. I wasn't too sure what was going on.

Next morning I was told that I was no longer second on the surgery list, but last. I had no option but to accept all this, and I still felt that, since we had prayed about the decision, if there were changes, there were probably good reasons for them. I waited, somewhat anxiously, for my turn.

At some point around this time, I was visited by a member of the chaplaincy team. I expressed some of my anxieties and asked if we could pray together. I had noticed that, though she visited each person in the room, she had not prayed with the others, and I knew that I needed prayer. I had asked her if she would kindly arrange for someone from the Roman Catholic community to bring me Holy Communion on Sunday, should I still be there, and she had said she would do so. Now, when I asked for prayer, she said, 'I'm not a Roman Catholic. Does that matter?' I told her that I didn't think it mattered to God, so why should it matter to us? Apparently, the situation had come up before, in the line of her duties, and to some people, it *had* mattered. Well, they missed out then, because she prayed with me beautifully and I was very grateful. I also wondered if seeing this made an impact on the other people in the ward… God works in mysterious ways…

The other ladies in the side ward were very pleasant company. All were, I think, older than me, but when you are all down to basics, in bed and in night-clothes, it is the inner person that you see, not their age or station. They were all 'legs', and I believe all had skin grafts over wounds that had failed to heal, but each lady was very different. One was quite a private person. She was happy to converse from time to time, read a great deal but volunteered almost no information about herself. She was caring, noting the needs of others, but also, I believe, happy to be solitary. After a while, she was deemed well enough to go home…later, the bed was occupied by another.

The second lady was also good company, but profoundly deaf. It was obviously very difficult for her to be in that situation. Sometimes she had to resort to a pen and paper in order to communicate with the doctors and nurses and on other occasions she would get the wrong end of the stick and might have appeared foolish, when in fact she was nothing of the kind. Her hearing aid had a tendency to whistle which sometimes kept the rest of us awake, while she slept on, oblivious. On one occasion, a nurse tried to tell her that it was making rather a racket (it being about one in the morning) but she didn't understand, and, as the aid was lost down the bed, it was not possible to silence it! This lady was sadly, in some ways, very cut off. Despite the efforts we made to include her, it was very difficult for her to follow small talk and she slept a great deal. Perhaps I could and should have done more… I learnt in conversing with her that she had recently endured a great deal of personal tragedy. Her cross was a heavy one, for sure, yet she was always warm, friendly and concerned.

The third lady, though elderly and at this point inactive, was sprightly, usually a keen walker and was excited about her plans for the future. The new place she was moving to sounded great, and she was often surrounded by concerned family members, of whom she was clearly very proud, and rightly so. She had the bed opposite mine, and we learnt much about each other. I hope that she enjoyed my company as much as I did hers. I was able to render some small service to her, in that she complained that she always forgot to ask the nurses the questions she had meant to recall in their presence. We discussed from time to time things that she had wanted to ask, and I did my best to make a mental note of them and jog her memory at the right time. I believe this was helpful and I hope she had no objections, though I don't believe she did, because she gave me a book to bring away when I was discharged. She was a sweetheart.

Having been nil by mouth from midnight in preparation for my surgery, I was visited mid-morning by the anaesthetist who would be responsible for me. He asked me about my response to anaesthetics and listened when I told him that whatever I had been given for the very last surgery I had undergone seemed to have suited me very well. He said that he would check the notes and aim to give me the same concoction. He also said that, since I wouldn't be going down for a few hours, I could have some water, which he personally brought me. I was very grateful for this small act of kindness, as I had in fact asked a nurse if I might drink a drop of water at about seven that morning, and she had said I could not. It is important to remember here that the nurse could only respond as the doctors told her to, for fear of being disciplined otherwise, but the anaesthetist was, in a sense, his own boss, and so free to make a decision based on his knowledge.

Sometime after mid-day, in the early afternoon, I went to theatre. The lady who took me down had done so before, and so we chatted, and, as before, she labelled my spectacles so that I could keep them for comfort, but they wouldn't get lost once they came off. A junior nurse, who had been told that she might watch the operation if I was willing and had asked for my permission to do so, also came with us. She was disappointed that I had been pushed back on the list, as she knew that this meant she would have to go off duty part way through the procedure. The fact that she would leave this ward next day made this her last chance and she had really been looking forward to it. Once down at the theatres, a further disappointment awaited her, because, although we had been told that the senior nurse had cleared her visit with the theatre staff, the sister in charge said that nobody had asked *her*, and the young lady might not go in; she could stay while the anaesthetic was administered, but after that, she must leave. This, I felt, seemed rather harsh, and I was disappointed on the young nurse's behalf.

Administering the anaesthetic was something of a nightmare, due once again to my rotten veins! I tried not to mind, watching the two poor guys in the theatre anteroom wince as they stuck the needle in again and again, without finding a suitable vein. I believe it was some time between the fourth and the sixth attempts that my tears began to flow and I could not stop them. It sounds so childish, because this really was a very small needle, but it really hurt. Part of the problem was the need to try for veins in the back of my bony hand, rather than for those in my nice, plump arm, but basically, the chemotherapy has messed up the lot – maybe for life? I don't know. I prayed a lot, silently. The anaesthetists were clearly as distressed as I was. They said that, no matter how long you do this job, and no matter how many people you have to stick needles into, it never becomes any easier to inflict pain. I could tell they were having as hard a time as I was. One of them made a remark about what to do when I eventually would lose consciousness – something about luck, or picking a dream or a thought, I don't recall – and I told him that the last thought at that point is always the same one: 'Here we go, Lord.'

It was on the seventh attempt that the vein was successfully hit and mercifully, very soon after that, came the expected sensation of 'going under', mentally committing myself to the care of God, because, once inside that theatre, I would be in His hands, under the skills of those He had appointed for my care. It seems to me that when such a time comes, total abandonment to the Lord is really the only sensible course of action.

I awoke in post-op. recovery, feeling cold. The attendant nurse fitted me up with one of those plastic over blankets that fill with hot air. Wonderful! I drifted, and then became aware of the need to empty my bladder. They obligingly provided a bedpan, but my muscles refused to respond to the promptings of my nerves – nothing doing! I had to settle to living with the discomfort, and, in due course, was returned to the ward.

I did not feel nearly as bad as I had expected to. I was not allowed out of bed, but I felt no sickness, and, drifting in and out of a doze, was able to converse between times with the others. I was again provided with a bedpan; by now, my muscles were responding, and oh, the relief! At the evening drug round, I took the prescribed medication: two paracetamol to keep pain at bay, one large dose of ibuprofen to act as anti-inflammatory and two Erythromycin tablets as covering antibiotics against infection. (Penicillin would have been more normal, and kinder to the stomach, but I am allergic.) When Martin came to see me that night, bringing food, I ate two-thirds of the meal he had provided, and I enjoyed it.

This next account I include because I feel it reflects the vulnerability of being a hospital patient in a ward full of strangers, and the need for, perhaps, more sensitive handling of private matters than sometimes occurs...

It was in the middle of the night that I had to call once more for the bedpan. To my horror, I found that I had lost proper bowel control, just as had happened after my major operation for the double DIEP flaps. The medication was probably responsible, playing havoc with my digestive system... I cleaned myself up with wipes, and informed the nurse, who said that, should this happen again, it would be necessary to obtain a specimen, just in case we were dealing with some nasty bug. Like most people, I guess, I hate this kind of thing with a passion. Because of the requirement for a sample, when I again needed the toilet next day, I had to use a commode at the bedside. In any case, this was my first time out of bed since anaesthetic, so I doubt if I would have been permitted to walk to the bathroom.

I asked the nurse, who had drawn the curtains around my bed, to open the window, feeling very uncomfortable and self-conscious. She did so, and I used the commode provided. As clearly as if spoken beside me, I heard one of the other patients say, 'What *is* that stink?!' Mortified, I asked the nurse to tell the lady concerned that I apologised for the 'stink' but it was beyond my control – I could do nothing about it. The nurse took the commode away to obtain the sample, and I went back to my bed, but I didn't want to look the others in the ward in the eye.

I am convinced that the lady who had spoken so frankly had not known what was going on, and had not meant to cause awkwardness or offence. Neither had I! Her consciousness of having spoken out of turn and my consciousness of having been the cause of it, meant that neither of us was at first able to relax back into the friendly banter that had been exchanged before. At first, we could not even make eye contact, and the others in the ward, aware of the charged atmosphere, felt equally ill at ease. If any nurses ever read this account, may I make a plea for you to offer to transfer your patient, wheeling them on the commode before you remove the seat, to the privacy of a bathroom in circumstances such as these? Apart from anything else, I'm convinced that episodes like this one persuade the other patients that the last thing they will ever do is expose *themselves* to the same vulnerability. Therefore, they simply don't 'go' until they are able to walk to a bathroom, yet the members of the medical staff are constantly asking them if they have had their bowels open! Surely this is a counter-productive situation for all concerned? There is much talk, these days, of maintaining privacy and dignity. Maybe a little forward thinking could have helped…

The irony of all of the above is that I was visited during the day by doctors and a lady from pharmacy, all of whom cautioned me that the drugs I was taking were famous for 'going right through you.' The consultant who had done the surgery proposed a change of antibiotic, but I refused. I was convinced that my problems had been caused by taking the medication on an empty stomach, and I was also afraid that, if the medication was messed about, I'd be at risk of infection. After all, it had been after a similar episode, and when my antibiotics were stopped, that infections had set into my wound sites before, and I still bear the scars. Though the medication upset my stomach for the duration, the acute problem did indeed cease once I was eating regularly.

On this day after the operation, the first doctor to visit was the consultant who had performed the surgery. He was pleased with my progress and, aside from the discussion I mentioned above regarding the antibiotics, generally very satisfied. Seeing my family photograph (which I had asked Martin to bring in for me) at the bedside, he asked about it. We are not, as I have mentioned before, a typical family in some ways. My complex heritage is Anglo/Irish/Welsh/Spanish/Jewish/Afro-Colombian, Martin has distinctive Celtic colouring and may be part Romany, Liz, adopted at the age of three months, is Anglo/Irish/ West Indian, and Dan, adopted at three weeks, is Afro/French by heritage. In short, we are the family that God put together, in a very real sense, and our own version of the United Nations to boot! My African consultant was clearly delighted to learn this and went away saying, 'I can see you are a Christian!' Well, if that is so, it is only because of the goodness and generosity of God, seen in my life; I, a barren woman, have two wonderful children, gifted to me and to my warm and loving husband by the Almighty – and by their brave and generous birth mothers who refused to destroy them, but bore them and then painfully parted from them, to give them a chance of normal family life. We are daily grateful to God, and to these courageous, strong women.

Perhaps, in the end, this is what the whole scenario of my cancer, its treatment, and the subsequent reconstruction has been about. Throughout these events I, and others around me, have seen the goodness of God at work in my life, His generosity, in both small ways and great – my lollipops from the Lord! – His care and His power. God did not give me cancer, but He allowed these events to take place that I, and those who have travelled this road with me, might understand His goodness and draw closer to Him. It is paradoxical to think of how much I have gained from some pretty devastating experiences – but the mind of God *is* mystery, and the mind of Helen is not capable of comprehending it, but can stand in awe and gratitude before it!

When the consultant had left, another doctor came to see me; the one who had seen me first after my admission on this occasion. Smooth, tanned and handsome, he was appropriately professional but he alarmed me greatly by telling me that I would need further surgery because my breasts were still too unequal. Remember, at this point, I was recovering from surgery only the day before, which was supposed to be the 'final shot'! I told him that, and he said that he knew, but that I appeared to have very little swelling to resolve and a marked difference between the sizes of my breasts, (this I could see for myself) hence his conclusion.

Throughout that day, I stared obsessively down at my breast. I phoned my husband and bewailed my situation. I phoned my dad and did the same. I visited the bathroom, now that I was allowed out of bed, and opened up my nightshirt, trying to examine myself through the dressings. I stood front on, and in left and right profiles. Most of all, I worried and fretted, particularly as I really didn't want to risk, once again, all the complications attendant upon surgery.

One of the nurses, seeing my distress, told a senior nurse what had happened. Later that day, on two separate occasions, senior nurses came to counsel me. Both agreed with the doctor that there was a great disparity remaining. One told me that both she and her daughter had a great difference between their left and right breasts but, when pressed, she said she felt that my situation was more extreme than theirs. She went on, however, to contextualise this problem by pointing out to me the great number of things I had to thank God for, compared to which this was a minor setback. At this point, I was also offered the help of a professional counsellor, but I refused. After all, if there is a physical problem to resolve, no matter how much you talk about it, it remains. I had been visited by the counsellor the last time I was in hospital. She is a lovely and very helpful lady, but at that point she had concluded that my disappointment, apprehension and frustration were justified emotions in the circumstances. I could not see how things could be any different now.

When my friends visited in the afternoon, I told them what this doctor had said. I was absorbed with the problem, really, despite their generous gifts of sliced melon, which we shared, and fruit salad, which I kept for tea, and even the warmth and love which they delivered with their gifts. This was a really difficult day for me.

A small amount of 'light relief' was provided when the time came for the mandatory night-time injection of a drug to prevent blood clots. Most often, this injection is given into the stomach. The nurse tried, with little success, to gather up some fat into which to inject. She said, 'I like to get a good handful, but you haven't got much, have you?' I replied, 'No, because it's all on my chest now!' and we began to giggle, at which point, waving the needle wildly in the air, she complained, 'I can't do this while you're laughing!' Actually, by this time everyone in the side ward was laughing, but there you go…

The next morning, I again saw the consultant who had done my surgery, with another doctor who often accompanied him. I told them what had been said and how depressed I felt, and they asked questions to ascertain who it was that had said these things to me. I was concerned, and said that the young doctor had not said anything untoward about the consultant, but they reassured me that they were only trying to establish whether the medic concerned was sufficiently experienced to make such a judgement, and, having established who it was, they determined that he was not.

Patiently they explained that this doctor had been wrong about the issue of swelling; that, after the extent of surgery that I had undergone, there would *always* be swelling, and that the swelling would not be fully resolved for three, or even six, months. Only after this period would we know whether further surgery was necessary. The surgeon explained that he had been concerned about the possibility of removing too much tissue without realising it, so that, once the swelling subsided, there was a problem in trying to balance an over-adjustment. He told me that the consultant I had originally been under had visited him towards the end of my surgery and had been very happy with what he saw. He reminded me of something which I already knew; no woman has equal breasts. Bra manufacturers, he said, take that into account. He felt certain that I would be able to purchase underwear that would give a reasonable fit on both sides. When these two gentlemen left, I felt a whole lot better.

Much later, I was visited by my previous consultant, who echoed much of what the other doctors had said. He said, 'It is bigger; no doubt about that, but until the swelling is resolved, it is impossible to make any decisions. I don't think you will need anything else done, but, if you do, it will only be something very small, under local anaesthetic. I think it will be possible for you to buy a bra to fit.' I was much comforted by all of this. With the dressings removed for the surgeons to look more closely at my breasts, I had been able to see that all of the hard, lumpy tissue, which had resulted from the earlier fat necrosis and had led me to describe my right breast as a 'potato', had now gone, as had some very ugly scarring. The whole area looked much more natural and much less ugly.

When the doctors had gone, one of the nurses came and asked me if I had a bra with me. I told her I only had one which I had worn to come in; that I had planned to go home in a camisole with a little built-in support, because I knew the old bra wouldn't fit after the surgery. Moreover, the bra had one of my 'foam friends' stitched into the left cup. She took the bra and deftly cut out the little prosthesis, and then put the bra onto me, to show me that it was now too big in *both* cups, thus, I *had* benefited from the surgery. With the bra in place, despite the poor fit, my shape was better, and the difference less marked. I was encouraged to wear it to support the healing breasts, and I felt more confident once I did so.

During this same day, as I have mentioned before, one of the ladies on the ward had been discharged, and now another, also a 'leg', was wheeled in to take her bed, but this lady was clearly not at ease. She had come that morning to outpatients to have her leg dressed, and been sent up to the ward by the staff down there, because they felt that her injury would not resolve without a graft. Gradually it emerged that this lady lived with a little dog for company, which had been alone indoors since early that morning, because she had expected to be back home long since. Also, it became clear that, having had little experience of hospitals, she was not surprisingly very apprehensive, experiencing that sense of loss of control over one's fate which I know only too well. In the end, it was agreed that she would go home and 'put things in order', returning next day, and this she did. My friends kindly wheeled her back down to the car park, and she drove herself away.

The next day she returned, with a friend for moral support. Clearly calmer, she chatted to the rest of us in the ward, and we warmed to her immediately. She showed me a really interesting embroidery technique she was using on a piece she was working to while away the time, and I showed her how to work the bedside T.V. and telephone facility, and one or two other things besides. The trade-off worked very well. It also served to remind me that, for many, a trip into hospital can be a devastating experience. Unused to anything about their surroundings, thrown in amongst strangers, in a totally alien environment, people are often disorientated, anxious and very insecure – who wouldn't be?

We had seen a clear demonstration of this from another source over the past few days. On our ward there were bays of four beds, but these were usually 'women's bays' or 'men's bays' so that the only time we were in mixed sexes was on the main corridors, heading for the shared facilities. An elderly man had been admitted at the same time as me, and he was allocated a bed in the next bay. He was a lovely, gentle man, but so completely disorientated that he frequently wandered into our all-female bay looking for his bed and had to be steered back to it. We became accustomed to redirecting him, and, over time, he began to recognise his environment better and would say, 'I'm in the wrong place again, aren't I?'

I suppose hospital is a place where you may expect to be reminded of other people's problems. Sometimes this can happen in unexpected ways. I was familiar with the difficulties of people who are tobacco dependent in this environment. There are notices in all the bathrooms forbidding smoking, and the poor souls have to take the lift down to the ground floor and snatch a crafty, draughty fag near the entrance. I understand the dangers of smoking and applaud the hospital's decision not to permit it, but I can't help feeling sorry also for those deprived of their 'prop' when they are sick and in an alien environment. I had, however, never thought, before this latest visit to hospital, of how it must be to one whose dependency is alcohol…

I went one evening to the toilet and was struck immediately by the smell of beer. Beside the lavatory pan there was a spillage of drying ale, in which the plastic four-ring structure, which keeps four cans together for a multiple purchase, was lying. There was no evidence of the cans themselves; presumably they were buried in the bin. One can only speculate on the loneliness and desperation of the person who perhaps obtains the beer from a visitor covertly, then locks themself into a toilet to drink the contents of all four cans as quickly as possible and at once, spilling the precious beer in their desperation to do so. There is always someone whose problems are worse than your own…

I had originally been told to expect three days in hospital and two weeks convalescent at home. Admitted on Wednesday, I had had my surgery on Thursday, and had been seen by two medical teams on Friday, who decided that the drains inserted into my wounds should be checked again on Saturday. On Saturday it was determined that one of the drains could be removed, but in fact it was not, because no nurse came to do the job (none seeming to be available), and I was eventually told that it would be O.K. for another day. The other drain, with its vacuum bottle, was determined to be too productive to remove at this point. I was anxious not to stay in hospital any longer than I had to, due to my very great fear of infection, so the surgeon at one point said to me, 'Well, you can go home with your drain, if you want to, and come back to have it removed,' but I didn't find this prospect at all appealing.

Eventually, it was decided to leave the drain in place, but 'de-vac' it. Later, on Saturday evening, the consultant I had originally been under came by, and gave instructions to 're-vac' the drain…

On Sunday morning, I was delighted to note that the drain contained well under ten millilitres, usually a sign that it was due for removal, but the nurse warned me not to get my hopes up, as the contents of both bottle and tube were still very bloody. Usually a drain comes out when the fluid in the tube is running straw-coloured. However, when the doctor came, he deemed that the drain could come out, and, standing at my bedside in his Sunday morning 'civvies', began to pull the adhesive dressing away from the wound on the right breast. I took a deep breath and said, 'Doctor, I don't want to teach my grandmother to suck eggs, but…' I never managed to say, 'Have you washed your hands?' because he immediately said, 'I'll just wash my hands and get some gloves.' I knew I was probably speaking out of turn, but I also knew only too well all the setbacks that infection can cause, and I was taking *no* risks this time!

Anyway, he examined me thoroughly, and pronounced me fit to leave. I was delighted. I tried and tried to call home, but the phone was permanently engaged. I rang my husband's mobile and got the answering service. I rang the home phone and the mobile again. Eventually, I got through to Martin, and the poor man told me that he'd taken the phone off the hook to be sure of a little peace in the bathroom! I think he felt like a constant information service for much of the time I was in hospital, because of the family members who were eager for updates.

Martin said he'd be there to fetch me as soon as he could, and I set about dressing and clearing out the contents of my locker. Once dressed, I felt like the proverbial fish out of water on the ward. I was eager now to leave. The nurses sorted out the medications I needed to take home with me – at least a few more days of anti-inflammatory drugs, and a full further *week* of the antibiotics! Yuk! I was told to take the pills as prescribed, and to keep a watch on my temperature for the next few days. I was also told to remove my dressings after two days and make sure that 'nothing nasty' was happening underneath them. Just before lunchtime, I said my goodbyes to my companions of the last few days, whose company I had really enjoyed. One of them, knowing my great concern over my uneven bosom, looked at me critically and said, 'Well, a blind man'd like to know the difference!' Much cheered, I left with Martin.

I was quite pleased because, now that I was 'out', I would be able to attend mass that evening in one of our local churches. On the ward, we had asked if there was a Sunday service in the hospital chapel. At least one of the other ladies would have been eager to attend, had there been one. We had also asked if there would be a Christian service broadcast on the hospital radio – at this time there was one in the hospital in my hometown. (Sadly, I believe it has now been forced to close down.) A young male nurse had gone off to find out for us. On returning, he told us that there was no service in the chapel on Sundays, and nothing of that nature would be broadcast on the hospital radio. However, Communion would be brought to us, if we so wished. I had told him that I had already asked for a member of the chaplaincy team to bring me Communion. (They let me down, in fact, on this occasion. By the time I left, no one had arrived, and I believe Eucharistic ministers always come in the morning...) I felt sorry, however, for the others. At least one lady there had a need that was not met. She had never been confirmed, she said, so did not want Communion, but would have liked to go to church. She was obviously shy regarding a personal visit for prayer by one of the chaplaincy team, so she got nothing at all. Vulnerable as she was, and detained in hospital – indeed bed-ridden at that point – I think this was a great pity.

Martin and I had a snack lunch and a quiet afternoon, went to church in the evening (where I sat throughout the mass) and cooked a meal late, upon our return. I settled into convalescent mode. From time to time, I felt fraudulent. I was so much better than I had been on the previous occasion, and I had not been instructed as to anything I was forbidden to do. Occasionally, as when I tried a little ironing, I found my limits, having to stop before I had finished the job I set out to do. Also, I did not attempt to drive, since doing so soon after a general anaesthetic can invalidate insurance cover.

The main concern, I guess, was to protect my fresh wounds and give them a proper chance to heal. The sutures this time were soluble, and very neat. Left to heal properly, they would give a very good result. Had I returned to work too soon, there was always the chance of a knock, or in a worst-case scenario, the possibility that I would have to intervene between fighting students. Such events occur rarely, but they do happen, and it would have been disastrous if such a thing had undone the surgeon's good work.

I monitored my temperature for a few days as instructed, and, on the Tuesday, looked under the dressings with trepidation. No problem, no redness, no bleeding! I had been warned that some heavy bleeding was possible from the site of the drain, but even this did not occur. I had been told that I could shower any time from the Thursday onwards, but I didn't risk it, preferring to continue to strip-wash.

Meanwhile, I busied myself with getting hold of some bras that would fit. I phoned up two mastectomy suppliers, on the basis that they would be used to fitting problem chests, and explained to each that, upon measuring, I had discovered that there was a difference of one cup-size between my two breasts. I gave my size, and asked them to send me underwear to try; anything which they felt might give a suitable fit. Then I waited.

When the parcels came, I eagerly tried on all that had been sent. True mastectomy wear proved impossible to try on, because the pocketed cups, even when stretchy, did not 'give' back to the bra lining. I was told that ladies often remove the pockets, but it is, of course, necessary to buy the bra if you do that, and that seems a rather pointless and expensive exercise if you don't know it will fit... I gave up on these items. Of all that had been sent to me, from two different firms, only one bra was really suitable. Not quite a perfect fit, it was certainly a passable one, with a little to spare at the front of the left cup. Best of all, it was made in very pretty lace and available in black, white and ivory, with matching briefs. I sent back the rest, and ordered more sets of this item, only to discover that the model was discontinued... In fact, I was able to obtain enough to kit me out for the next six months, but what would I do then, I wondered?

I had reason to ponder. I had been told I would have to wait at least three months to be able to see the final outcome of this last round of surgery. In the meantime, my unequal frontage showed a good deal in some things, and less in others. Oddly, clothes that fitted closely were better than loose garments, where the hang of the item tended to accentuate the problem. I wasn't sure how noticeable this disparity would be to others, when I began to just 'dress and go' once more. Clearly, I was going to have to wait and see, and pray about the time when I would have to make any decisions. In the meantime, my aunt once more spoke to me on the phone. Still full of concern for me, she told me that she was sure that, however disfigured I had been, Martin and the children would rather have me alive, than dead from MRSA. She went on to tell me that she had been anxious because she personally knew four people who had died from the infection. I understood this entirely. Every time I contemplate being cut for any reason, the thought of serious infection is at the forefront of my mind. Remember that, at the time when this conversation took place, I was monitoring my temperature and checking underneath my dressings, fearful of ominous changes.

It was a full thirteen days before I dared to remove the steri-strips and risk a shower. It would have been at least a day later than that, had I not attempted to tackle a very dusty job indoors, (admittedly in bite-size pieces – you do not go mad at any job when convalescent!) and felt mucky afterwards. I held my breath as the strips came off, and looked very closely at the wound sites as I showered, but only a pin-prick sized piece of the scar was unhealed, and even that did not bleed; it was just a bit pink. I had come through without any signs of infection this time, and only now, when I realised how well I was, following the latest surgery, did I really understand how very ill I had been, following the last bout.

When my follow-up appointment came through, it was for the day *after* my planned return to work. I phoned the surgeon's secretary, who promised to call me back if he felt that resuming teaching presented any problem. Meanwhile, I attended my six-monthly call-back appointment with the oncologist. He examined me and seemed to be very pleased with my progress. For belts and braces purposes he ordered x-rays of my spine and pelvis, (since I'd had some backache) and a blood test, but he made it clear that he did not expect these to show 'anything out of the ordinary'.

Famous last words! I really should have been used to this by now, but in fact I was really thrown by what happened next. The oncologist had told me that, if I had heard nothing from him in seven to ten days, I could consider myself in the clear. He added that, after ten days, I could telephone his secretary if I felt I needed to, just to be sure, because she would have the results. Me being me, I duly did so, and was told that she had no results to give me, but would check with the oncologist. A little later, having still heard nothing, I called again. The blood test, she said, had been fine. She would speak with the doctor that same day and get back to me about the rest. She called back later. The doctor, she told me, would like to see me in clinic on Thursday.

Scary stuff! – And I told her so! Could I not, I pleaded, be added to the Wednesday clinic, so as to avoid an anxious wait..? She would check... No, the doctor wished to have time to speak with me properly and if I was tacked onto the earlier clinic we would be rushed. – Help! Scary was fast becoming panic stations. This *must* mean there was something dodgy on the x-ray, since the blood test had been fine. Did I have a secondary cancerous lesion in my lower back?

It is a form of torture, really, this waiting game. Some people have little trouble in believing they are fine until told otherwise. I am not one of them! I could not live without my faith, but have to admit that sometimes, on such occasions, I am still full of fear, at least between times. The Thursday appointment was a long time coming.

When finally I got there, the oncologist was both frank and kind. He acknowledged the level of my fear, apologised for not allowing me to come to the earlier clinic, told me that he was sorry that this was happening to me of all people, since he knew it must have made me anxious, and explained that we still had no clear result, because there were some shadows on my x-ray. 'What,' I wanted to shout, 'are you telling me, and what does this MEAN?!'

Patiently, he went on to explain that it was very common to find shadows on x-rays of the pelvic area. Often, he told me, they were due to nothing more sinister than gas in the bowel, which the rays cannot pass through. The problem was we could not be sure without further tests, and with my history... There it was again – another 'but in your case'! How this syndrome had dogged me from the start of all this!

He ordered a bone scan, and I now know, because my husband assures me that this is so, he ordered an MRI scan at the same time, but it is significant that I just somehow failed to register this at all. I do remember telling him that my back pain came and went; that it was almost non-existent on that particular day; that I thought it would be much worse if it was due to cancer; that I would expect to have gas in the bowel on a morning x-ray taken after a high fibre breakfast, and that I thought this was by far the most likely explanation. He said he would happily go with that until results of tests showed him otherwise, but he did not cancel the tests! I went home to await appointments in the mail. I remember arguing vehemently with Martin when he told my friends I was to have an MRI scan as well as the bone scan. I was sure the doctor had not ordered one.

In due course, the appointment for the bone scan came through. On the given date, I first went to work. As I arrived, my mobile phone rang. It was the hospital. 'Don't say you've called to cancel,' I pleaded. No, they were asking me to attend earlier. That was going to be difficult, as I had arranged cover for the rest of the day but promised to be in at the start. I did a little juggling, and I went for it. I would only have been able to be in the centre where I teach for that first part of the morning anyway, because, once injected, I was radioactive and therefore not allowed to sit close to children for any length of time. I had the jab and then went home until my call back time of around one o'clock, when I was scanned.

In the waiting room, before the first injection, I shared the space with a little girl of around three years old and her parents. Dressed in 'Barbie' and sparkles, she was a delight. She had been to the children's ward already that morning to have a canula inserted under anaesthetic, so that her injection would not be painful. Watching her, talking to her, put things into perspective for me. Even if my results were undesirable, I'd had a good life, so far. What had she had, by comparison, and what was she doing here? I could not ask. I had to be content to wonder.

The scan itself was easier than the one I had previously been through, after my initial treatment for cancer. Somehow, the young lady in charge put me more at ease. Also, I knew better this time than to try to read anything into the manner of this gentle, cheerful person. I had tried that on the previous occasion and only succeeded in frightening myself half to death! This time, I was more relaxed and I didn't leave my jewellery behind when I left! Before leaving, I was advised to make an appointment with the oncologist, two weeks after, for the results. As soon as I got home, I did so. I knew that this would be the appointment that would set my mind at rest...or not.

Oh, 'the best laid plans...' A day or two later, an envelope landed on the mat inviting me for an MRI scan. Martin told me that yes, he'd been sure the oncologist had mentioned this. I was devastated, because I had been equally certain that he had not! I was really upset. It was obvious from the date given that it would be pointless to attend for the appointment I had arranged for my other results. I phoned the oncologist's long-suffering secretary, who took advice and made me another appointment, much later than the first. My period of anxiety was not to be so quickly overcome!

During this testing (in more ways than one!) period, God was walking at my side. Christian friends, especially those at the 'Verbum Dei' community at the end of our road, understood my level of stress and did not berate me for it. God's timing is pretty wonderful, too, for it just so happened that, during this time, we had a visit to the parish from the ministry of Fr. John Campoli, an American priest, who brings his healing ministry to our shores annually, and also a wonderful parish mission, led by Miles Dempsey, down from Liverpool for the purpose. I was so covered in, and surrounded by, prayer. Our kindly parish priest also understood my fears and prayed over me. Isn't it wonderful how God uses those around us to ease our distress? I suppose, in truth, I should not think it at all remarkable that there was so much support around, just when I needed it.

The MRI scan was, in some ways not at all related to medicine, an unusual experience. On arrival, I was told that the lady in the waiting room, who had the earlier appointment, had not yet been called in because the scan room was in total darkness and they were waiting for a technician, who had been called to replace a fuse. A little anxious about whether I would reach work by the time I had promised to arrive, I settled beside this lady to wait. As you would expect, we got to chatting. Strange how sometimes, in talking to a total stranger, you very quickly get into some quite deep stuff. Anyhow, this lady was very thirsty, and, seeing a water fountain but no cups, I went round to ask the receptionist if she might have a drink, and I guess that, to some extent, broke the ice.

My companion was from South Africa. I do not, even now, really know her views on the apartheid regime that used to be in place there. We talked a little about the country, and I told her that I would, perhaps, have liked to visit, but had always felt that it might be difficult, since we are a mixed-heritage family. I produced photographs to prove my point, and she told me that there were still some places where, yes, things would be difficult; others where it would be less so.

The receptionist was keeping us posted from time to time, but the technician had still not arrived, so we continued to converse. Discussing why we needed our scans, she learned of my cancer and was plainly very curious about the reconstruction. There comes a point where just talking about something is futile, so I whipped my sweater up and showed her the surgeon's work. She was both interested, and admiring of the skill. She also felt it remarkable that I looked so very well after all I had been through. I told her about God's goodness to me. I don't know where she stood on such matters, but she did not seem to disagree. The thing about all this is, we would never have had this conversation – and I certainly wouldn't have 'whipped up my sweater' – if we hadn't been thus stranded by a technical fault. I don't believe that any such conversation is an accident. I know that I admired this lady for her calm and controlled manner in a time that must have been anxious, and also for talking frankly about some things that may have been difficult for her. Perhaps she also took something beneficial away from our conversation. Who knows?

Still no technician, and the receptionist, plainly worried about getting so far behind schedule, asked tentatively if either of us would be prepared to be scanned in the dark. She explained that there would be light in the tube itself, but not in the room.

My companion was not happy at the thought of this, so I offered to go ahead, on the principle that I could always come out if I bottled it! Removing anything metallic and clothing with metal fasteners, I went in.

I had never had an MRI scan before, and had only a sketchy idea of what to expect. A kind of bed was made for me on a platform at the mouth of the tube, and I lay down and was covered with a blanket. When ready, I was moved up inside the tube. This was a very claustrophobic experience, the 'ceiling' of the tube not being very far above my face, but the white interior of the tube was lit (and in fact the room lighting itself had been repaired whilst I was being set up) and there was a grille above my head through which I could hear the voices of those organising my scan. Through this medium, I was constantly advised of what to expect: different noises, scans of different lengths, a movement of the 'bed' inside the tube and so on. For my part, I had simply to lie extremely still for between fifteen and twenty minutes. They were, it is true, very noisy minutes, and some of those noises eerily disturbing and uncomfortably loud, but I was prepared in advance every time and was never unduly alarmed. I was very grateful to the medical staff responsible, for their careful and considerate handling of me throughout.

Once the scan was completed, I dressed and left. Nothing is ever, as I have observed, quite straightforward. I discovered as I was dressing, that the left earpiece of my specs was broken at the hinge, beyond repair. It therefore became necessary, since I cannot manage without glasses, to go from the hospital to the opticians, where, after a fruitless search for another frame to accommodate my lenses, an inspired young lady technician 'cannibalised' an earpiece from a pair of designer specs, fitted it to mine, and charged me the princely sum of a fiver! A bit different from the hundred the new frames would have cost, had they fitted! Believe it or not, after everything, I arrived at work at the time I had planned to, and all was well.

My 'results appointment' was now to be in the week before Christmas. I was not, during this period, unduly worried. I had been covered, as I have told you, in prayer from so many sources, and my backache came and went, varying in intensity, which made me believe it could not be due to cancer. When the day came, Martin and I went to the hospital and sat, as you do, apprehensively in the row of chairs in the corridor, awaiting our turn. We chatted a little to those waiting with us, one of whom turned out to be the daughter of a lovely man I know through church. There was another patient between this one and myself, so our chance to chat was, sadly, limited. I had known through her father of this lady's history and would have enjoyed getting to know her better.

The lady on my right I did not know at all, but she seemed happy to talk. She pointed out to me something in a magazine that she had been reading. I cannot remember exactly what it said, but I know it was about death, and she said some things related to how people cope with the death of a loved one. We discussed coping mechanisms a bit – a strange conversation for the queue of a cancer clinic, and I felt that some other people within earshot were not terribly comfortable with this, so I allowed that conversation to peter out. Then my new companion asked about my medical history, and I told her my background in brief. Emboldened by her empathetic responses, 'Yes, I had all that as well,' I went on to ask why she was there. Her reply really shocked me. What a brave lady she was, and how inspired I was by her courage!

She had leukaemia, she told me, and it could not be cured; only palliatively treated to give her as much time as possible.

I gathered, from her reluctance to tell me how this had come about, that it was a side effect of her treatment for cancer, and I have since found out that this is indeed so. A very small proportion of patients treated with Epirubicin during their chemo (which cuts your chances of recurrence of cancer by one third) do go on to develop leukaemia. Epirubicin's potential benefits far outweigh the potential risk, so the drug is routinely given where it is warranted. This lady had been *so* unfortunate – and she knew it. To have gone from breast cancer to this, and to know that it was the treatment for one that begot the other!

She told me that she had known since Monday – it was now Thursday – and had come to terms with it. I asked her if she would mind if the prayer group prayed for her, and she said she would be delighted. We have. I thank God for this chance meeting with such a lovely person. She and her husband were full of plans to make quality family time from this point on. Their focus seemed to be completely on making happy times for those they loved. May those times have been truly blessed for these beautiful people!

These days, when I see the oncologist, it is usually not the consultant whose name heads up the clinic that I see, but another, younger man, and we have grown more familiar with each other over time. He did not so much invite me in on this occasion, as sweep me off the corridor with a, 'Come on then!' to which I replied, 'Woof!'

Once inside the consulting room, he told me good news. The bone scan and the MRI were both normal. I do have deterioration in my lumbar spine and a thickening in my sternum, both, most probably, due to age, but he could discover no changes that were cancer related. What a Christmas present!

The shadows on the x-rays were due to nothing more sinister than gas in the bowel after all!

Thank goodness this consultant has a good sense of humour. He finished the consultation by saying that he didn't want to see me for six months, and that he didn't feel the slightly crusted mole on my neck (which I slipped in for a quick check) was cause for concern, but that I should keep an eye on it. My husband, not given to reverence, then said, 'So to sum up, it was gas on the x-rays, her other problems are due to age, and she's to keep an eye on a crusty mole. Would you say that means my wife is a crusty old fart?' Men laugh together at these kinds of things, don't they? I didn't dignify it with a response!

Christmas, a good one, a *family* one (not always possible once the fledglings have flown the nest) came and went, and singing around in my head along with the carols was, 'I don't have cancer in my spine!' It was the extra gift that I hugged to myself throughout the season.

We did indeed sing carols: we sang them around the wards of the local hospital, where some of the nursing staff recognised me, we sang them in church, and we sang them in the home of my friend, the midwife and nurse who had accompanied so much of my cancer journey. The gathering at her house was special. Our mutual Chinese friend was home from her new job in China for a few weeks at this time, and because her house in Harlow was now rented out, was staying with Martin and myself. A whole bunch of us now gathered at Gemma's to give others a chance to spend time with May, to eat Chinese takeaway, (cooked by our good friend Jimmy, whose wife I had met in the ward when I was going through my first surgeries to remove the tumour) and to celebrate the birth of Jesus by singing carols accompanied on guitars.

Christmas Day itself had been spent at home – just Martin and myself and our two children, our lodger friend having been invited elsewhere. Such intimate family time is so precious now that our children each have their own address. We were both very grateful for the fact that they spent the day with us, and came to Birmingham with us the next day to see the extended family. But Christmas can't last forever.

For some time it has been a kind of tradition in our household that, after Christmas, Martin takes me to London, to the sales. Usually, he either treats me to a little something that catches the eye, or gives me some 'mad money' to spend. The hidden agenda is a visit for him to Harrods's toy department, followed by a little shopping in their food hall!

This time, there was a sort of second hidden agenda. Martin had decided to buy me some pretty new underwear, so that I would feel good about myself.

We went to all the usual good department stores, and I started out enthusiastically enough, rummaging through the lingerie, picking up items that I thought may be worth a try… but I became increasingly downcast, as time wore on, because I found nothing approaching a fit. One store informed us that their fitting specialist did not start work until the afternoon. In another, an attentive lady spent a considerable amount of time with me, before declaring that there was too much difference between my breast sizes for her to be able to fit me successfully, and asking me whether my surgeon was going to give me a reconstruction! I wanted to scream, 'Lady, this is the Rolls Royce of reconstruction! You're looking at it!' And I wanted to cry. In fact, as the afternoon wore on, I *did* cry. Poor Martin was very fed up. Here he was, trying to do this thing to please me, and I was progressively 'going down the tubes'. The whole plan

was, as they say, going pear shaped. It might have been easier if
my breasts had, too!

Eventually, in one of the stores, I found two very pretty
basques on sale, which had moulded, pre-formed cups. It
didn't seem to matter in these that one side was a bit too big
and the other a bit too small, so we bought them, and some
matching briefs, and honour was satisfied – but I was left with a
problem. After all, basques are not what I call everyday lingerie,
and you may remember that I had bought up the entire stock
of the bra that had fitted me, supplied by the mastectomy
specialist, because the style was discontinued. (The fitter lady
had said in any case that she considered this more of a crop-
top, though I didn't agree). What was I going to do next time I
needed underwear, if the cream of the London stores couldn't
help me? This was really depressing, because, it seemed, I had
been fooling myself in believing that perhaps I was more-or-
less sorted, and wouldn't need further surgery. The only light
on the horizon was that the surgeon had definitely told me that,
if I needed any further intervention, it could be done under
local anaesthetic. Clearly I had some hard thinking to do.

So January brought the hospital appointment with my
plastic surgery consultant. When the young lady at reception had
written the time down for me at the end of my previous visit,
I had expressed surprise and pleasure, as it was late in the day
and I would not have to miss work to keep it. As the date drew
closer, Martin became apprehensive about his ability to attend
the appointment with me, and it turned out that he was right
to be so, because the firm that employs him insisted that every
employee must attend a tutorial day on 'risk assessment', with
no exceptions, and would not release him from this obligation
so that he could accompany me, even if it only meant leaving
early. What about *my* risks? Who was going to help me to assess

them? Going alone also worried me because, as I have said before, the hospital is at a distance, and my sense of direction is notoriously bad!

On the day itself, I went to work armed with route instructions, since I would go directly to the hospital from work. A few people suggested that, since this seemed to be a late clinic, perhaps I should just ring and check. Thank God in His goodness that I did! The receptionist had clearly written 5.30. What she *should* have written was 15.30! Rapidly, I set about arranging to leave early, grateful once more for my accommodating employers.

I made the journey there more easily than I expected. The thing is, when you are driving to a hospital appointment your mind has other things to occupy it than merely reading the road, but, distractions not withstanding, I got there in good time – and spent *ages* looking for a parking space, beginning to feel that, after all the planning, I might still miss the appointment! I asked God to find me a space, and He came up trumps!

I did not have to wait very long before I was called. It was the usual routine – undress to the waist, put on a theatre gown, fastened at the front – but the man who came in to see me was a complete stranger. He was a consultant, and very pleasant indeed, but he was neither the doctor whose clinic I was under, nor the man who had performed my most recent surgery. This was the call-back appointment to discover whether further surgery would be needed, and it seemed a little odd to have a new man on the case.

I showed him my chest. I talked him through the difficulty I had had in trying to buy underwear. I explained that I had been told that the difference would not be enough to be a problem – and he suggested an implant! Hey! The only reasons that I

had been referred to the plastic surgeon in the first place were
that I had been very unhappy with the lack of symmetry on
my chest, unwilling to wear external prostheses, and *dead* set
against implants. So here I was, post surgery, being told again
that an implant was my way forward – and no Martin by my
side. I told this gentle man a little of what I felt. He talked of
waiting anyway; said that he wouldn't consider further surgery
until the last had settled for 12-18 months. Hadn't I had my
surgery only last May? Yes, I told him, and further surgery in
September which was supposed to be the end of it all! (Except
for nipple reconstruction, and how could you do that on very
uneven breasts? You'd end up with a chest that looked cross-
eyed!)

The doctor talked about how the surgery I had already had
was a miracle in itself. He reminded me of all of the things
that could have gone wrong. He said that, instead of feeling
frustrated, I should give thanks to God. He said that there was
still lots they could do for me. Eventually, he asked if I would
like to wait to see my original consultant, who was currently in
theatre.

I returned to the waiting room. The nurse had realised
just what an ordeal this was becoming and asked another to
make me a cup of tea, since the refreshment booth was closed.
I sipped gratefully and waited.

My consultant appeared, in surgical scrubs. Back I went
(same routine again) and waited until he had spoken with his
colleague and the nurse. Both men then came in to see me.
My consultant now said that he had no doubt that it was very
difficult for me to buy underwear. He could see there was a
big difference. I think he, too, was disappointed at this state of
affairs. He agreed with his colleague that, for the best cosmetic
outcome, I should be given an implant.

I couldn't believe this! Hadn't a young doctor, who had been working alongside him the first time I had been in this very hospital, told me that the great thing about my surgery was that I'd be *all me* at the end of it? Hadn't this kind man himself told me, before discharging me last time, that I would be able to buy bras to fit – and that, *if* I needed anything doing, it could be done under local anaesthetic? (I feel certain now that, at the time, he had believed this.) Now I was being told that I needed to come in for a surgical implant. I reminded him that I had been offered implants as an alternative to this transplant reconstruction right at the outset, by a previous hospital. He said that they would never have been able to fit them successfully under such a thin layer of skin as I had had. Fair enough, but they obviously hadn't known that when they'd made the offer, and if I hadn't wanted implants then, why would I want them now? He said that I had an unreasonable prejudice against implants. He said that, if I wished, they could make the right breast smaller instead, but that would be a bigger job, involving the removal of about ten ounces of tissue. He said that they might be able to do that under local, if I could tolerate it. (That didn't sound good.) He told me to go away and think about it. I did.

Firstly, and probably unreasonably, I felt betrayed. Why had he told me before I left hospital that, when the swelling passed, the difference would be manageable? (The answer, of course, is that he thought it would…) Secondly, he had visited the theatre during my last operation. Why had he not suggested removing more tissue then, and spared me all of this? (Now, of course, I feel certain there were good surgical reasons.) Thirdly, he knew from the start that I hadn't wanted any implants. Whether or not their use had been possible initially was really a 'red herring'.

Gradually, as I drove home, certain things began to dawn on me. I had never asked him for breasts. That had been his suggestion. What I had asked for, had been symmetry, and that remained as far away as ever, though the appearance of my chest was dramatically improved. And when he *had* spoken about breasts, I had made it clear that I'd be happy with 'two fried eggs'. Even my smaller breast was no way a 'fried egg'. I felt that, just maybe, there was another consideration here. My excellent surgeon had worked terribly hard, through a delicate twelve-hour procedure, to graft tissue – a lot of tissue – onto my poor, decimated chest. Perhaps he just wasn't comfortable now to be asked to remove yet more of it? Gradually, I formulated a forward plan. It was the only thing to do, given my state of mind. If you just go over and over things in your head, you go nuts.

I would do five things.

I would research implants again, using the Internet. I would see whether the statistics relating to implant failure had improved. Perhaps he was right. Perhaps my attitude *was* unreasonable.

I would lose some weight. I did not really need to do this, but I needed to know how a change in my body weight would affect my new boobs. This was in case, after all the problems I'd had with fat necrosis, there were actually substantially different numbers of fat cells on the two sides of my chest. Would the difference between my boobs be greater or less with weight loss? (I guess I could have tried weight *gain* but hey, there are limits!) I would make a real effort at the gym, alongside the weight watching, and see what a little 'body sculpting' would do.

After losing the weight, I would go to *the* bra shop – Rigby and Peller in London. I would talk to their fitter and find out whether it was possible to find underwear that would fit without a struggle. Remember, despite the difference, I was not at this stage 'packing' at all. What you saw was what you got, and most people just didn't know there was a problem, as long as I dressed carefully, though it is true to say that everything still had a tendency to 'walk to the right'.

I would write a letter to the consultant, expressing all of my fears, asking all of the questions that I wanted to ask, outlining my feelings. I would put *everything* into that letter, and I would not expect him to reply in writing, but to be ready to talk to me about all of those things when we had another consultation. I would have to think very carefully indeed about that letter!

Lastly (but really firstly and most importantly) I would pray for guidance, over and over again. Such an issue is not simple. Many people live with disfigurement through accident, fire, amputation and the like, and they just get on with it. But if they were offered a chance of improvement, and if they had a practical problem that could be improved, like mine over the underwear, would they then decide to live with it, or would they 'go for it'? And risks. No surgery is risk free. I knew what infection could do. Suppose I had further surgery, liked the shape, and then had to watch it all go wrong due to a raging infection? I felt that previous general anaesthetics had done my memory no favours. Was I ready for another? If the surgeon was willing to operate under local, could I bear it? I'd seen some pretty nasty things when they took away my navel that way! I would just have to try to seek out the will of God in all this. There are times when a direct line would be more than handy!

I didn't have a direct line, but I did have the prayer group at Barking, and I was there very soon after all of this happened. Terry had prepared readings for the evening. To my amazement, one of them was the passage from Jeremiah which has followed me all the way through this experience, popping up time and time again –'I know the plans I have for you, says the Lord; plans to prosper you and not to harm you. Plans to give you hope and a future.' I felt, when I heard this, that at least the Lord was still in there with me. I would just have to learn to listen really well: you know, 'Speak, Lord, your servant is listening', not, as was all too often the case in my prayer, 'Listen, Lord, your servant is speaking'!

Not long after this decision-making process, I got onto the Internet and looked up implants, surfing sites, some of which belonged to the manufacturers and suppliers. Many women, I know, are happy and trouble free with this solution, but I did not like the information I found one bit! I made notes for my letter to the surgeon, and decided that, for me, implants were still 'out'.

I set about trying to lose weight. This is not easy when you are not really overweight but within the normal range. Still, I knew a loss of around five pounds would do me no harm, and I had a tendency towards 'love handles' that might be nipped in the bud, so it could be a good plan! I did fine for a few weeks, and dropped around three pounds, but at this point I caught a truly lousy and persistent cold. If I was to be able to speak, I had to suck lozenges, and I don't do sugar free, because free from sugar usually means full of chemical nasties, so the weight slowly crept back up and I had to start all over again. At least these things teach the art of persistence...

I visited *the* bra shop. The staff members there are especially well trained and will give you a private fitting by appointment. You can have bespoke bras made for you. However, *I* wanted to be able to buy off the peg, because whatever way I went about buying underwear now was going to have to be sustainable for the rest of my life… And affordable! For me, this was not going to be the solution.

In the event you know, having tried prayerfully to explore options, sometimes you just have to bite the bullet. My surgeon reluctantly accepted from my outpourings that I was not going to be able to live in peace with an implant; I would always be anxious about how it was behaving. He agreed to another surgical reduction of the right breast. To him, this must have seemed something of a travesty: before the cancer, I had been a 34H bra size and I believe his mission (not mine) had been to restore me to my former self as far as possible; now I was asking for that hard-won tissue grafting work to be messed about yet again… I was booked in once again for surgery (much less major than anything previous, it is true) and we set about it.

I had been told, you will recall, that this last adjustment could be done under a local anaesthetic, but it was not to be. I had another general – and I woke up with better symmetry than I'd known for years! The hospital took photographs. It's not (but whose bosom is?) perfect; my right breast is still larger than my left, and I know for a fact that my long-suffering surgeon is *not* going to shave any more off it! But part of the problem always was that the left breast had unavoidably been re-sutured to irradiated skin after the major infections I suffered at the initial surgery. Consequently, it has some scar tissue that does not move as freely as normal breast tissue, due to the repairs it has undergone. This can accentuate the deficit – and nobody is to blame.

This, then, was it. This was the last major 'do'. And this left me with a perfectly respectable 36D bust (I never did quite beat the 'love handles'), but best of all, I could walk into Marks and Spencer or British Home Stores and buy a bra! Lots of bras in fact! Can you believe it? I'd always had to take even my pre-cancer, over-large bosom to specialist shops and spend big money on big lingerie, yet now I could behave like a kid in a sweet shop! Alleluia!

And we could have just left it at that. I was well and I had boobs and they almost matched. Many women have natural boobs with a greater disparity between their sizes than mine. I had and I have, no desire to undergo further surgery on that front (pardon the pun), but I didn't have *nipples*! Mine had, almost seven years ago, gone off into the incinerator, and now, at my discharge appointment following my final breast size adjustment, I was being asked if I'd like some. Just like that. 'Have you considered nipple reconstruction? We do find that our ladies feel it gives closure.' I had thought about it. I didn't know much about it, except that it involved tattoos... I was definitely interested...

Now, my breasts are good. Of course, I'm a map of scars, and my cleavage is a little untidy (which happens when double mastectomies are reconstructed, because the central line is sometimes fudged by scarring). I avoid low plunges, for this reason, but otherwise, I feel I look good. However, at the point when this question was asked, the answer seemed obvious. We'd all come so far together: God, me, my family and my boobs. Why not finish the job? How hard can it be?

Nipple construction is fascinating. Imagine a cross with the bottom stick missing, or an upside down 'T'. That's how the cuts were made. Three small rectangular strips of still attached tissue, all cut and raised from the point where the nipple needs to be (and this is calculated, measured and marked, using stats from thousands of female bodies). The surgeons suture the donor areas from which the rectangles have been lifted and then craft these living strips together in such a way as to create a raised area that really looks like a nipple. I had had some sensate tissue – a small area which still had breast sensitivity – on my right side, but it was not exactly where the nipple would be constructed. The nipples, of course, had to be sited to give the optimum cosmetic result; nobody wants 'wall-eyed' boobs! The surgeon said I shouldn't be too concerned; I probably wouldn't lose this sensation, as the donor area of skin would come from the area of my breast which had feeling. I felt I was on the pathway and had to trust my guides. They seemed to be very well versed in what they were doing.

They did great, but *I* made one mistake. I opted to have this procedure under local anaesthetic. (I think I had, by now, had fourteen general anaesthetics in my life to date and I felt that was enough). The members of the surgical team were universally kind and considerate throughout the operation, but it *was* gruelling and I felt cold, shivery and shell-shocked afterwards. If *you* are going for this, have the general and wake up cosy…

After the operation, the new nipples are huge, but they will shrink mightily and must be protected while they heal, so special dressings are applied. I had known about this but I still wasn't prepared for the experience of proudly bearing two facsimiles of 'SpongeBob SquarePants', one on the front of each breast – I kid you not; bright yellow, and with a hole for the new nipple in the centre of each!

Straight after the surgery I went to relax in the day unit and was duly discharged after an hour or so and several cups of tea. During the healing period, I had one scare, when one of the suture lines opened a little, after the soluble stitches dissolved. But it was not, in the end, significant... On that day, when we phoned for advice, the hospital asked me to drop in so that the team could check me over. I was allowed to leave with the wound duly creamed (with an eye ointment!) and dressed and go straight to friends in London for tea as planned. We were only about an hour late!

Nipples, of course, have colour and this is achieved, as I mentioned, by using tattoos. Nurses trained in the art match the colour they will be using to the skin-tones and lips of the patient and skilfully blend pigments, keeping careful records of exactly what proportions of what pigments they have used in the mix. Once all of the surgical parts of the nipple reconstruction were successfully healed, I attended, by appointment, to get *my* tattoos.

It is fascinating to be asked how big you would like the areola to be! I hadn't thought about it... I didn't know... I'd be guided by them, as they see a lot of women... Thankfully, the nurses were brilliant. The colour sorted, they used an instrument which is a little like a very small version of the head of an electric toothbrush, but with tiny needles instead of bristles, and worked the pigment into the appropriate area – Not, I was told, a perfect circle, because that doesn't happen in nature and it would look strange.

The procedure makes the area bleed, and that mixture of blood and pigment has to be allowed to dry and scab. The scab must not, under *any* circumstances be picked, or the tattoo will not 'take'. Over a period of about ten days, the scab sheds naturally and after this, the patient attends for a call-back appointment to see if anything further needs to be done. In my case, it didn't. I was finished. Done.

The amazing thing is, now that I have nipples as the normal focal points of my breasts, everything else looks so much better. Friends are curious. They ask, could they possibly have a peek? They are amazed at how good my chest looks. Some are even envious (but then they remember how I got here). My surgeon said, 'Well, it's not the best we've ever done, but…' and he was clearly pretty pleased with the overall outcome. He had been so very patient and understanding with me for so very long. One friend more recently commented that I 'could almost do topless'; not that I'm planning to, but at fifty-six at the time she spoke the words that was quite a compliment. I am happy to this day that I travelled to the appropriate end of the road and I know that I did the right thing. We got there… And I will always owe so very much to so very many people…

I do still have some sensitivity, some feeling, in my right breast, but many of my reconstructed sisters will tell you that they don't. My left breast lacks sensation, but that's the side where much of the pectoral muscle was removed and the site of my radiotherapy, so that's not surprising. For some very lucky ladies I have heard that the appropriate nerves have been spotted by surgeons during surgery and spliced into position as a bonus. I guess it's a bit of a lottery, but, if so, I am content with my lot. I swim in a carefully chosen bikini and change in public changing rooms without embarrassment, and that has to be quite a result for someone with my story. (However, I divert for a moment just to say chlorine is best avoided by those with nipple tattoos – It can fade them over time and if this happens they may need to be re-done, hence the need to keep such careful records on pigments.)

A small jump forward in time now. At the time of this incident I have been 'whole' for about a year, I guess. The normal rhythm of life and work has resumed; in fact I'm very busy because somewhere in the middle of all of this I have achieved a promotion. I am walking (a longish walk, which I like to do regularly) up the main road at the top of the town, towards home. I may well have been coming from an evening meeting at church, but I can't be certain. It's high summer and the ending of a very warm day, sun still seemingly direct at around eight-thirty, so I sling my jacket over my shoulder and walk in jeans and T-shirt. And something happens that ought to make me blush. A car full of men in their twenties or early thirties goes by, with all the windows open, due to the heat. One of the occupants yells at me from the window: 'Get 'em out!' He's suggesting, somewhat lewdly, that I remove my T-shirt. Strangely, I feel no offence. All I want to do is giggle. If only he knew!

I look back over my fears and thoughts described in Part One, at the start of this journey. I have so very many reasons to be grateful... I am still supported by my loving, extended family. I continue to teach (semi-retired now) and to enjoy my working role. My 'journey' has, if anything, enhanced my effectiveness within this, gifting me with greater empathy. I am still so much a part of a supportive church family. The pattern of the music ministry within that has changed, but my level of involvement has not; my vocal range has also changed, but I still have (and am frequently asked to use!) my singing voice. My body has **totally** changed, it seems, through so many phases, both in appearance and in chemistry, but I'm happy living in it! My self confidence is intact; I feel just as much a whole, attractive and sexually capable person as before, and my (our!) marriage remains strong. So do the many friendships on which I have leant for support throughout my travels, some of which I would never have known...

My faith in God has been strengthened; paradoxically, having lost so many 'bits of me' along the way, I am so much more healed, so much more whole, though still travelling... Still also in receipt of the 'lollipops' from the Lord that remind me that He is still walking with me. This was and is the story of a route; only God can decide when I've arrived...

If you have been travelling with me a while, I thank you for your company... and wish you well on *your* road...